Cremation and Urn-Burial; or, The Cemeteries of the Future

W. Robinson

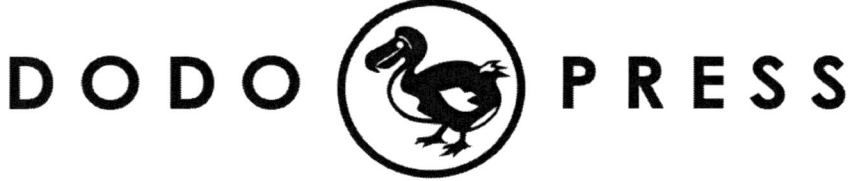

CREMATION AND URN-BURIAL

OR

THE CEMETERIES OF THE FUTURE

BY

W.ROBINSON

1889

CREMATION AND URN-BURIAL.

THE sanitary reasons for preferring urn-burial are strong, even by those who, for other reasons, are not among its advocates. I propose to consider the subject from another point of view - the aesthetic one, or that of the beauty of nature and art, which an improved system of burial would make possible in all that relates to the resting-place of the dead. Many are apt to consider cremation as meaning the absence of all the forms of respect we usually bestow on this; and finally, of such associations as are generally gathered round the spot. But it is, on the contrary, the present system of burial which is open to the greatest objections in this respect. The history of many graveyards in crowded cities is this: Comparatively few years' accumulation of bodies, say from one to two generations, then finally closing from overcrowding. A generation or two passes away; many changes occur among those interested in preserving the graves, and soon their voice is heard no more in the matter. Then, at the will of some one or more persons desirous of disposing of a place which, frequently, is extremely valuable, at any moment the remains of every person buried therein are liable to be subjected to the utmost degradation; to be carted away as secretly as may be by some contractor, whose only object is to find a convenient shoot for them. Such changes are not unfrequent in London, though they are usually carried out as quietly as possible.*

* DESECRATION OF CITY GRAVEYARDS.-Are we not becoming too much accustomed to the idea that anything, however sacred, may be turned into money? Is not this the case with regard to burial-grounds? They fetch a large sum and they disappear. After the Great Fire of London care appears to have been taken in rebuilding the City to reserve in the main the burial-grounds of the parishes in which the churches themselves were not rebuilt. They are dotted as green spots all over the City, as many must often have observed. When the present extensive buildings of the Bank of England were erected, one whole parish was swallowed up. It was generally understood that its churchyard was respected, and is represented by the pleasant open garden court which gives such cheerfulness to the

offices around it. St. Clement Danes' parish appears to view the subject in another light, and makes short work of the matter. Some years ago one of its burial-grounds, situate in Portugal Street, was disposed of for the site of part of King's College Hospital, and all trace of its former use has now disappeared. We have just heard that it has parted with another of its burial-grounds, adjoining Clement's Inn, for the site of a portion of the New Law Courts. One burial-ground, its principal one, in the middle of which the church of St. Clement Danes stands, still remains to the parish. An effort is being made, in connection with the Law Courts, to induce the parishioners to sell this also. Can we hope, after what has been done, that they will be proof against it? I trust we may. Sites can be got without invading these small churchyards, which have been bought over and over again by those who lie in them.-W. B., in *Times.*

That secrecy, however, is not always exercised in operations of this kind is evident, from the fact that the remains from a disused cemetery in the west-central district of London were spread over a couple of acres of Kensington Gardens a few years ago.

In Paris the state of things is no better, as there the bones are taken out of the ground, and the headstones and other memorials often destroyed within a few years of their being placed in position.

In America, owing to the extent of the beautiful cemeteries now existing near the larger cities, such evils are not so apparent, though they exist there also. No matter how large cemeteries are, they are certain, in time, to have serious drawbacks from the conditions inherent to the present mode of burial.

Under this system, the whole area of the place must, sooner or later, be filled with bodies, and must, eventually, be closed, unless in very sparsely-peopled districts. The small cemeteries in a city like London disappear from time to time, as noted above. The park-like ones in America may seem more secure from violation; but every future generation cannot, as the present one, enclose many hundreds of acres of valuable ground for burials. The American way is more decent than what is usual in France, but the difficulties of space alone would make it, if not impossible, a difficult plan to follow in the future.

BEAUTIFUL CEMETERIES POSSIBLE WITH URN-BURIAL.

WITH an inoffensive and prompt system of reducing the body to ashes, this drawback of our burial system at once disappears. The ground not being occupied with bodies, there is no need to close the cemetery at any time. In graveyards of the size of the present overcrowded London ones, urn-burial could be carried on for hundreds of years without the slightest offence to the living. By the common consent of mankind "God's acre" is most fittingly arranged as a garden; and as the place for urn-burials need not occupy more than a fourth of the space of a large cemetery, the whole central or main part would be free space for gardens and groves of trees. The cemetery of the future must not only be a garden in the best sense of the word, but the most beautiful and best cared-for of all gardens. But as the present way of using the ground often leaves no room for either garden or planting, it may be best first to consider the subject in relation to monumental art, and to the dismal regiments of stones which cover the soil of our graveyards.

It is impossible to over-rate the opportunities for improvement in all that concerns the beauty or even the sentiment of the matter, which would be secured by the condition of *permanence.* Apart altogether from the closing of the burying-place, the decay from exposure, which now defaces memorial stones, is a very serious drawback. So recent a headstone record even as that of Gilbert White, in Selborne churchyard, is found with difficulty by the stranger; and many memorials erected in London cemeteries during the past fifty years are now crumbling to dust. There is no reason why these stone records should not be at least as enduring and as legible as the paper ones within the church. Most persons will agree that it is desirable that they should be so; now they are the very image of decay. While long duration is not possible under our present system, with urn-burial the simplest stone inscription may be in as good order a thousand years hence as today. With it also there would be a satisfactory realisation of the meaning conveyed by the word cemetery-a resting-place, or place of sleep, for the dead.

THE PRESENT GRAVEYARD NOT A PLACE OF REST.

The ordinary city graveyard being now only of temporary use, such monuments as it possesses share the general fate of all the other materials when it is closed. The frequent disturbance of the ground for interments is against any good work in such art as the place invites. In a London cemetery, such as that on the high road near the Marble Arch (St. George's, Hanover Square), it may be noticed that the memorial stones are crumbling away, although this is one of the best cared-for of closed cemeteries. One cannot regret the poverty of the "art" displayed in such places to decay and be forgotten. In Paris the foundations of roads are made of headstones only a few years erected; and though in London memorial stones, erected to "perpetuate" the memory of persons, are not cleared away so promptly, the result in the end is very much the same. Pieces of broken monumental stones, some of them bearing dates, were among the *débris* for which a contractor found a convenient place in a London public park. The effect of the tombs and stones dotted thickly over crowded city cemeteries is as ugly as it can well be, but it is in accord with the very temporary interest which, in the nature of things, these places have for the public.

Notwithstanding the great attention and vast and unselfish expense devoted by the American people to their cemeteries, this passage, from Oliver Wendell Holmes, points to the fact that the same evil exists there:-

"The most accursed act of vandalism ever committed within my knowledge was the uprooting of the ancient gravestones in three, at least, of our city burial-grounds, and one, at least, just outside the city, and planting them in rows to suit the taste for symmetry of the perpetrators. The stones have been shuffled about like chessmen, and nothing short of the Day of Judgment will tell whose dust lies beneath any of those records, meant by affection to mark one small spot as sacred to some cherished memory. Shame! shame! shame !- that is all I can say. It was on public thoroughfares, under the eye of authority, that this infamy was enacted. I should like to see the gravestones which have been disturbed or removed, and the ground levelled, leaving the flat tombstones; epitaphs were never famous for truth, but the old reproach of 'Here *lies*' never had such a wholesale illustration as in these outraged burial-places, where the stone does lie above, and the bones do not lie beneath.

NOBLE AND ENDURING ART MADE POSSIBLE THROUGH URN-BURIAL.

By the adoption of urn-burial all that relates to the artistic embellishment of a cemetery would be at once placed on a very different footing. One of the larger burial-grounds now closed, perforce, in a less time than that of an ordinary life, would accommodate a like number of burials on an im-proved system for many ages. The neglect and desecration of the resting-place of the dead inherent to the present system would give place to unremitting and loving care, for the simple reason that each living generation would be as much interested in the preservation of the cemetery as those that had gone before were at any previous time in its history. We should at once have-what is so much to be desired from artistic and other points of view - a permanent resting-place for our dead. With this would come the certainty that any memorials erected to their memory would be carefully preserved in the coming years, and free from the sacrilege ·and neglect so often seen. Hence an incentive to art which might be not unworthy of such places. The knowledge that our cemeteries would be sacred-would be sacred to all, and jealously preserved by all, through the coming generations-would effect much in this new field for artistic effort. In days when careful attention is bestowed upon the designs of trifling details of our houses, it is to be hoped that we shall soon be ashamed of the present state of what should be the beautiful and unpolluted rest-garden of all that remains of those whom we have known, or loved, or honoured in life, or heard of in death as having lived not unworthy of their kind.

In endeavouring now to obtain any good effects, defeat is certain through the essential conditions of the present mode of burial. With urn-burial everything we can desire for the artist is not only possible but easily attained. Soft, green, undisturbed lawns; stately and beautiful trees in many forms; ground undisturbed, except in certain small parts; a background of surrounding groves; no hideous vistas of crowded stones; and the certainty that the monumental work done may remain permanently. And these are not all of the advantages which another system of burial would give us from the point of view of monumental art. The adoption of cremation does not necessarily do away with the tombs. So far from that, in old Roman cemeteries beautiful tombs may yet be seen, with the urns within them in as good order as when placed there two thousand years ago. In such cases a single tomb served as a family burial-place. The expense which is now spread over a variety of graves, headstones, and the purchase of ground would, intelligently applied, build a tomb which might endure for ages. To make it beautiful and enduring as man and stone could would be an aim not unworthy of an artist. A single burial in such an urn-tomb need not be so expensive as one in the commonest of the graves with which such large areas in our cities are now covered. The disturbance of the ground would not be necessary, as it is now; not to speak of the abolition of other onerous charges. The question of space is settled by the fact that one hundred of the simplest forms of urn could be placed in the space necessary for the burial of a single body in the ordinary way.

UGLINESS ABOLISHED AND INSCRIPTIONS AND MEMORIALS PRESERVED FROM DECAY.

THE need for headstones would be done away with at once by urn-burial, inasmuch as it would lead to burials in columbaria, which are, in fact, large urn-tombs. In many of them in Italy may still be seen exposed the little urns containing human ashes, dating from before the time of our era, in as perfect preservation as if placed there only a few days ago! Witness, for example, the marvellously well-preserved columbaria on the Vigna Codini and Via Aurelia. With our present system no trace now remains of some cemeteries in active, and as was supposed "permanent, use a few generations ago. The design of these columbaria or tomb-temples would be worthy of the best efforts of the architect, and their formation in the most lasting and noble form would not be so costly as the system of deep burial of the body, the headstones, and the continual and laborious moving of the ground. These buildings would save all memorials from destruction through exposure. This saving of all inscriptions and memorials of the dead from the ravages of time and weather is in itself a precious gain, which no one will undervalue who thinks of the importance of such records in legal and other questions of public or private interest.*

* The external history of the Etruscans, as there are no native chronicles extant, is to be gathered only from scattered notices in Greek and Roman writers. Their internal history, till of late years, was almost a blank; but by the continual accumulation of fresh facts it is now daily acquiring form and substance, and promises ere long to be as distinct and palpable as that of Egypt, Greece, or Rome. . . . We are indebted for most of this knowledge, not to musty records drawn from the oblivion of centuries, but to monumental remains-purer founts of historical truth-landmarks which, even when few and far between, are the surest guides across the expanse of distant ages-to the monuments which are still extant on the sites of the ancient cities of Etruria, or have been drawn from their cemeteries, and are stored in the museums of Italy and of Europe. The internal history of Etruria is written on the mighty walls of her cities, and on

other architectural monuments, on her roads, her sewers, her tunnels, but above all in her sepulchres; it is to be read on graven rocks, and on the painted walls of tombs; but its chief chronicles are inscribed on *steloe* or tombstones, on sarcophagi and cinerary urns.- Dennis, *Cities and Cemeteries of Etruria.*

Buildings, sacred or otherwise, may be adapted for urn-burial. The massive walls which should surround cemeteries might be formed into a covered way, or series of covered ways, in which urn-burial might be carried out.

ALL RELIGIOUS OR BEAUTIFUL CEREMONY EASY.

Inasmuch as no ceremony, sacred or otherwise, need be omitted in the mode of burial here advo-cated, so there would be fitting opportunities for the building of such religious structures as might be thought desirable in each case. When we come to the ceremony of urn-burial itself, we find it one that needs by no means be repulsive. The simplest urn ever made for the ashes of a Roman soldier is far more beautiful than the costly funeral trappings used in the most imposing burial pageant of modern times. Of urns of a more ambitious kind, the variety and the beauty are often remarkable, as may be seen in our national and various private collections. It would be a gain to art if some of the money spent on coffins, which rot unseen in the earth, were devoted to such urns, which do not decay, and which might be placed in the light of day, and perhaps teach a lesson in art as well as bear a record. There is a marble urn in the Woburn collection, with simple carving of the shoots of the common ivy over it, which is more suggestive of all that is beautiful in a memorial than any elaborate effort in a modern cemetery.

The ceremony of burial in this way, too, how different it may be made from that with which we are familiar! What a contrast there is between that picture of the noble Roman woman, surrounded by her maidens and friends, herself bearing her husband's ashes to the tomb, and the black array, the paid, half-besotted mutes, and the hideous box in which the remains of poor humanity are nailed up for a decay as needless as it is odious, to anyone who has seen it or thought of it! What a gain it would be to get rid of much of this Monster Funereal, the most impudent of the ghouls that haunt the path of progress! Vulgar show may, of course, be indulged in as much one way as the other; but it is pleasant to think of the ugly things and trades that may be abolished in cities when urn-burial became practicable. No doubt simplicity is possible, and is sometimes practised as far as may be, with the present system; but with urn-burial certain main causes of expenditure and show may be abolished altogether-great difficulties of transport being one of them.*

*I am speaking now of sentimental reasons, and I adduce a second, which first called my own attention to the unpleasant consequences which arise from our present system. It has been my misfortune to lose four of my nearest relations in different parts of the world. It has been also a subject of regret to me that their remains lie so far off. I care little for the fate which happens to their bodies; and yet, had such a. practice as cremation been in use, it would sometimes have been a comfort to feel that I had their ashes with me. Collected in an urn, they might either repose in columbaria, like those at Rome, or in a mortuary chapel in my own house.- The Rev. Brooke Lambert.

Given a crematorium near the town, and transport to the cemetery, however distant, involves little trouble. To a people scattered over the world, like our own, the ease with which remains could be brought from any distant country, without inconvenience and at little cost, to its final resting- place at home, deserves consideration.

BURIALS IN AND AROUND CHURCHES AND PUBLIC BUILDINGS MIGHT BE PRACTISED TO ANY EXTENT.

In connection with this part of the subject, it may be well to consider the opportunities which urn-burial would afford for depositing the inoffensive remains of the dead in our churches-old and new. It would have the great advantage of permitting burials to be carried out in churches and city graveyards to any extent and for any number of years. For various reasons, many persons would prefer burial in churches or near them; but, as is well known, the evils of the present system of burial became so horrible and so evidently dangerous in the case of city graveyards and churches, that burial within cities had to be forbidden by law, and not too soon. The state of things from which extramural burial saved us is again appearing in populous suburban districts. At Highgate, for example, strong undertakers' men have been made seriously ill while at work by the underflowing drainage from the higher parts of the burial-ground.*

* Communications have reached us, and observations been made, which compel us to draw serious attention to the con-dition of some of the cemeteries within the metropolitan district, which are rapidly becoming sources of peril not duly to the neighbourhoods in which they are situated, but to the whole metropolis. The emanations from some of the newly-opened graves are so horribly offensive as to occasion nausea among those who attend at funerals. As cases of actual illness, after being present at interments in some of the cemeteries, have occurred, there can be no doubt about the danger. Meanwhile the crowding of the graves is apparent. The number of bodies laid in the earth may not be excessive when calculated upon the whole acreage of the space licensed, but with an eye to the future the ground seems to be appropriated in parcels, while in some of the older cemeteries there is really no room for more graves, and the licence ought to be withdrawn. This is a matter of so much concern to the health of the community that we forbear to run the risk of weakening the evidence of facts by any comment. The intervention of the Secretary of State should not be delayed.-Lancet, September 27, 1879.

At no dis-tant day, under the present system, the numerous family tombs and graves in our extensive suburban cemeteries must fall into disuse. As extra-mural burial was not made law in London only, but in other large cities throughout the United Kingdom, it was a most radical change. Families who had for generations been buried in city churchyards have now to take their dead without the walls. Urn-burial would change all this. Establish this system, and people who have family tombs in our neglected city graveyards would begin to take a renewed interest in them, an interest that might save them from the desecration so often mentioned. It would tend to make our churches more interesting, and even our cities, for there is a certain fitness in men resting in death near the scene of their life and labours. The ashes of those who had deserved well of their country might be brought home from any distant place where they had perished, and receive a place of honour in our national churches' or buildings. Our great dead now, very properly, find a resting-place in Westminster Abbey, and there is no reason whatever why other great cities or other parts of the country should not have the same system for their own most worthy sons. But you cannot long have a place of horror and a place of honour too, and therefore urn-burial makes this public honour of the memory of the great dead to any extent, and for all time, not only possible but easy. Urn-burial is, in view of the change it would cause in this and in other ways, worthy in all its bearings of the serious consideration of the clergy. In the cemeteries of the future, of which a slight outline will be given further on, buildings will have to be formed for the reception of the memorials of the dead. In our churches these already exist, and would, for a long time, have the advantage over all others. Vaults, passages, niches, and walls would form suitable places for urns, and their accompanying inscriptions or memorials. In new or old churches, when these places were insufficient, portions of the building could be constructed for this purpose, which, being in complete harmony with the object and associations of religious buildings, would tend to encourage good architectural and artistic work. And not the church only, but the surrounding space would be valuable for the same reason. It is well to remember that some of the more beautiful tombs to be seen in modern cemeteries are based on ancient models of tombs, used as depositories for urns. Such family tombs would probably be built in our now disused churchyards; they might be above ground, and they would involve no disturbance of the earth, as the present grave-burials do, and little or no interference with trees or planting.

CEMETERIES BEAUTIFUL AND PERMANENT PUBLIC GARDENS.

Apart from the question of art is the important consideration of the great advantages the improved system would give us in adding natural beauty to the gardens of the dead, and improving many large open spaces in our cities of all sizes. Given a space equal to one of our largest London cemeteries, or one of those in America several hundred acres in extent, we may begin to outline what the cemetery of the future may easily be made. Permanent and inviolable it must be. The cemetery ~of the future not only prevents the need of occupying large areas of ground with decaying bodies, in a ratio increasing with the population and with time, but leaves ample space to spare for those open green lawns, without which no good natural effect is possible in such places. It is to be a national garden in the best sense; safe from violation as the *via sacra,* and having the added charms of pure air, trees, grass, and flowers. The open central lawns should always be preserved from the follies of the geometrical and stone gardeners, so as to secure freedom of view and air and a resting-place for the eye.

THE CEMETERY OF THE FUTURE: BUILDINGS.

Approaching the boundary, but not quite near it, should be erected a covered way, as strong and lasting as rock. This is to form a series of urn- receptacles on its inner side, well but simply designed. This alone, in the case of a large place, could easily be arranged to afford space for burials for ages. All other tombs and buildings of whatever kind should be confined to a belt of the ground within and near the covered way, and, with their accompanying groves, should not occupy more than a fourth of the whole space. The covered way should not be the work of one man or period, and, this being so, it would be well to separate its parts by planting or otherwise - occurring, if possible, in places commanding views of the surrounding country.

We are now considering a cemetery of the largest size and first importance - a national or metropolitan one. Several reasons determine that the covered way and main buildings shall not be on the extreme boundary; namely, to have them in as quiet a position as possible, as safe from injury on their outer as on their inner sides: to secure freedom from any kind of nuisance which might arise, from the buildings being placed too near property over which the governing body of the cemetery had no control; also to allow of the buildings being screened from the surrounding neighbourhood by tall trees, on any side where the views were not such as would add to the landscape beauty of the place.

Thus it would be possible to control the views not only from the centre to the covered way and tombs, and *vice versa,* but also beyond them, and to secure freedom from any objectionable sights or sounds. The actual boundary would be secured in a more ordinary but effectual manner. There being ample space within and without the great covered way and accompanying tombs for much noble tree-planting, the larger trees need not be planted near tombs, as there have been many instances of the disturbance of these by their roots. The buildings should be near and between groves of evergreens, and the dwarfer flowering, weeping, or columnar trees.

These would partly conceal and soften them, as seen from the central parts. A main walk passes by these groves and the monuments, and it should be the principal, and if possible the only, road in the place. A beautiful church or classic temple, such as that at Munich, might form the entrance; this and all other structures being built subject to the approval of a group of artists and architects who would see that their design and workmanship were not unworthy of the spot.

FREE AND SIMPLE BURIALS FOR THE POOR.

Some might claim the privilege of erecting urn- temples or other buildings for public use, or for securing free urn-burial to the poor who desired it. It may be easily shown that urn-burial is much the less costly way, and those who have to combat the prejudices against it must take care that it is made as inexpensive as possible. Moreover, as it is desirable that no person, however poor or friendless, who desires it should be denied for pecuniary reasons this mode of burial, so there should be free burials for the very poor - free from any demeaning condition.*

* The mode of burying paupers in London and Paris is an abomination and a disgrace. In London, as may be seen by reference to pp. 55 *et seq.* for the account of the Tooting Cemetery, it is a public danger as well as a horror.

Although the plan of this paper is to deal with only certain of the aspects of the question, not commonly considered, a very sad one which many must notice is that of the cruel sufferings of the poor owing to the ordinary system of burial. Few but those who go among them much know the hardships to which they are reduced through the death of the head, of the breadwinner, or other working member of the family. This is frequently preceded by the exhaustion of all the little means of the house, wholly derived, perhaps, from the labour of the one who lies dead. Then come these excessive burial and funeral charges, which often cannot be met, or, if met, absorb the last shilling in the house. A case was some time ago reported in the daily papers where an undertaker in London allowed a body to lie in the house till the police had to interfere, because the widow could not advance him the whole of the sum of eight pounds. Proportionate charges for the most useless and hideous of all forms of display are too well known in every rank; and cases such as the above are not uncommon in our towns, though seldom reported in the newspapers.*

* BOW STREET - AN UNBURIED BODY. - A poor woman named Laller applied to Mr. Vaughan on Tuesday, and stated that on Monday week her son had died. He was nineteen years old. The body was taken to an undertaker named France, who lived at 9 Great White Lion Street, Seven Dials, who agreed to bury it for £3 3s. She paid him £2 10s., but could not at present make up the remainder. The man France had made her sign a paper by which it was agreed that he need not bury the body unless the whole of the money was paid, and as she could not pay the 13s. the body still remained unburied. She had received only about £1 5s. Mr. Mitchell said the parish were quite willing to bury the body, but they had wanted the case to come before a magistrate first, as this was not the first case of the kind against this man France. He had been at this court and at Marlborough Street several times for not burying bodies.

SYLVAN AND FLORAL BEAUTY OF THE CEMETERY.

The sylvan charms of such a spot might be greater than is usually obtained in public gardens. The protecting architectural wall is far enough from the boundary to allow of groves of oak and other hardy native trees being planted outside it; these groves to have grass and wild and naturalised flowers beneath and between them. The interior groves and gardens might be the home of all the beautiful green things that grow in our climate. The main portion of the surface being always free for such ends, we should soon have a tree-garden which might even be of great public use. As some might desire to enrich the place with useful buildings, so others might claim to plant memorial trees or groups, where the opportunity existed. The views should be numerous and carefully considered. The planting should be wholly natural, in the best sense of the word. The outer portion, with its bordering tombs, columbaria, architectural covered way, and churches, should contain all the purely artistic adornments of the place; while the central portions should be quite free from the drill-master manner of arranging plants, and sundry like effects of a too prevalent style of gardening.

However all-sufficient the sylvan charms of the place might be, a desirable structure, in a bad climate like ours, would be the winter-garden, in which religious or burial ceremonies could take place at inclement seasons-in an agreeable temperature, and in the midst of a variety of beautiful living things. Few would object to this plan were it not from the objectionable way in which such structures are generally designed, the too frequent idea being that a glass shed more or less vast is the best plan. But the palm-house in the Edinburgh Botanic Garden, and a variety of structures used as winter gardens in continental cities, prove that vegetation thrives in buildings with stately and solid walls. Far more beautiful effects are obtained in such, from the contrast of the graceful forms of palms and other fine plants with noble building, than in the ordinary way. The temperature necessary to keep plants from temperate climes in health would be also that which would make it agreeable to people assisting at ceremonies, for which, of course, its most important spaces should be reserved.

CREMATORIUM, OR ANY STRUCTURE ANSWERING A LIKE END, BEST SEPARATED FROM THE CEMETERY.

As no body in a state of decay should ever enter into our garden-cemetery, the process of cremation, or any improvement on it, may be carried out else-where. But where, as will no doubt often be the case, the crematorium is constructed on the spot, it will be best to separate it from the general scene by planting or buildings. There is no reason why such a building should be so planned that any of its arrangements need offend the most sensitive person. There is no reason why any rite or act to be performed therein should not be carried out in accordance with due respect to every feeling of the friends of a deceased person. One of the earliest impediments in the way of improvement will probably be the failure to give due weight to these considerations in plans of crematoria.

An important result of the change herein advocated would be the preservation, as public gardens, of the many large cemeteries now in use, because with urn-burials continually going on they would remain inviolate. Their fate when filled and finally closed is, as before shown, very doubtful.

IMPROVEMENT IN PLANTING OLD GRAVEYARDS,

Apart from the question of improvement in burial, the present state of our rural cemeteries may be fittingly alluded to here. Possessing often considerable advantages as to site and soil, and associations that always seem to call for some care in adorning them with trees and flowers, they are often seen amidst our fairest landscapes as bare as a stoneyard, and, as regards vegetation, much less interesting than the hedgerows by which they are surrounded. The church-garden, even if small, need never be arid or ugly. But if there were only the walls-so often hard and naked-they alone might form a garden. Fresh foliage and blossoms are not often seen to greater advantage than against the worn stones of our churches, often unadorned with even ivy or Virginian creeper. Many of the best climbing roses and other climbers may be grown well on these walls. The several sides of the church might each have the plants suitable to their shelter or position. The walls round graveyards might also offer a suitable position for numerous low-climbing plants and bushes. Tombs may be partially garlanded with trailers, sweetbriar, or honeysuckle, and all this without disturbance of the ground or stones. It is best to adorn or gracefully relieve, instead of obliterating, such objects. The ground is generally well adapted for trees, and even the turf itself may be converted into a garden of early flowers. Indeed, the graveyard might often be a tree-garden, and one not without its uses. In planting it is essential not to hide the building from important points of view: too much care can hardly be paid to the views obtainable towards or from the site.

In cities and large towns trees often embellish the space round the churches to a much larger extent than in the rural districts, though the practice of planting evergreens in city churchyards is a foolish one in all ways, as they can only perish under our smoke plague. In such cases the summer-clad trees only should be used. Our old city churchyards could all be easily converted into oases of trees. The not unusual way of levelling or removing the headstones, and making the whole into a formal garden, is not the best. There is no real need for any sacrilege of the kind. The trees that flourish in such places are those that require little preparation of the ground-weeping and other native trees. Much short-lived and formal flower-gardening should be avoided, in consequence of the ceaseless care and cost it requires; the attention should mainly be devoted to the suitable hardy trees.

PRIVATE BURIAL-PLACES.

Near country seats urn-burial would lead to the family burial-place within the grounds-a quiet enclosed glade in some sunny spot, chosen for its beauty, embowered in a grove of evergreens, the grass sprinkled with hardy native or naturalised flowers only - so as to prevent any frequent attention on the part of workmen. Such a spot, with its carpet of turf, and walls of musical-leaved trees, wholly free from the long-lasting and many-staged horror of decomposition, which makes the ordinary churchyard so far from inviting to many persons, would form a fitting place of meditation for the living, as well as of repose for the ashes of the dead.

COUNTRY CEMETERIES.

The drawbacks of various kinds known to exist in connection with large urban cemeteries are often supposed not to exist in the case of rural ones; but, unhappily, they are sometimes in quite as bad a state as those in cities. Overcrowding is far from uncommon in country districts, but here there is less chance of the wholesale removals before mentioned. Some years ago, however, when certain changes in the church required the raising of a number of bodies in the churchyard at Cobham, in Surrey, the work of the navvies was of the most horrible and dangerous character, and was accomplished with difficulty in the early mornings, partly under the influence of repeated doses of gin administered to the men. Such removals are not uncommon, but they are performed as secretly as possible, for fear of raising opposition. In many quiet country places there is as great need to close the graveyard as ever existed in large ones, and sometimes greater danger, owing to imperfect drainage. In such cases any improvements or changes are extremely difficult to carry out, owing to the state of the ground. The same plan already spoken of in connection with great urban or national cemeteries would be proportionately no less advantageous, on a small scale, for country towns and villages. Danger to the living; pollution of earth or water; overcrowding; decay of memorials through exposure; hideous ugliness of stone, telling of accumulated horrors beneath the turf-all these, and many other evils, should be avoided in country as in town, while the various advantages of the improved system would be as precious in one case as in the other. The church and its vaults, and other unused spaces, and a covered way, replacing the whole or a portion of the usual fence, would, in most cases suffice for ages for urn-burial, leaving the whole of the churchyard itself free, as a beautifully planted spot. Urns placed under memorial windows, and in various positions on the walls, would invite monumental work of the highest class. The sentiment that people's ashes might repose in the church where they worshipped during life would not be interfered with in this case, whereas, frequently in rural districts nowadays, the present system compels the formation of a new graveyard away from the church.

THE "EARTH TO EARTH" SYSTEM.

The "earth to earth" system, or the burial of the body without a more or less solid covering, has been much talked of as a substitute for the usual mode of burial. It has in reality no merits whatever. By coffinless burial our ugly and noisome cemeteries can in no sense be bettered. The ground is occupied in the same way. It is an advantage to dispense with the needless and more or less costly wooden or leaden envelopes, but it is a mistake to suppose that very rapid decay takes place through their absence, as it has been proved that bodies deeply buried without coffins often decay slowly in ordinary soils. But even if the action of decomposition were always as rapid as it is in some soils, burial without coffins in no way frees us from the serious responsibility of needlessly polluting earth, air, and water. All the drawbacks, all the horrors, all the dangers of the present system would be just the same with this proposed alternative, which is, indeed, worthy of no serious attention as a substitute for the usual mode of burial. It has not even the merit of being a safe system, and those responsible for the public health could not permit of its use in the case of persons dying from confluent smallpox and putrid fevers.

This earth to earth system, so called, is merely a recurrence to the old-fashioned English way of burial in a shroud of woollen or other material. The wholly odious use of leaden coffins is defended by no one, not even the undertaker. Mr. Haden, who strenuously advocated the use of coffinless burial, with, as some have thought, the needless addition of basket- coffins, has dealt with this question in an ugly utilitarian way, which will, it is to be hoped, commend itself to few, and certainly to no one who has a particle of the feeling which animated the old Romans when they took their very effective precautions against disturbance of, or insult to, the ashes of their dead. It has been proved, over and over again, that the saturation of the soil by human remains is fraught with the greatest danger to the public health. We have it on the testimony of trustworthy and scientific witnesses, embodied in reports to Parliament, that disease on an extensive scale has been traced directly to this systematic and extensive pollution of the ground with bodies, yet Mr. Haden has nothing better to offer us than further pollution of the same description. I quote some of his reasons for his views. The italics are mine.

"Since," he says, "it is impossible for nature to err, and since it may be taken as an axiom that she will ever be found ready to supply us with the means of doing that which she requires us to do, need we ever be at a loss for ground in which to bury our dead? If it be true that a body, properly buried, is resolved in five, or at most six, years, it follows that at that interval, or at intervals as much longer as we please, we may *bury again and again in the same ground, with no other effect than to increase its substance and to raise its surface.* Is there, however, no ground in the immediate neighbourhood of our own city that would be the better for this increase and for being thus raised? The cremationists will tell us that there is not, but is there the shadow of a foundation for such a statement? Along the course of our great river from London to the sea, for instance, have we not vast lowland tracts of rich alluvial soil deposited by that very river and capable of being drained, planted, and beautified, in which, with equal benefit to the land and to ourselves, we may bury our dead for centuries? If, as we have seen, the surface of the Holborn Burial-ground was raised fifteen feet or eighteen feet by the interments within it of three centuries, *why should not the lowlands of Kent and Essex be raised and reclaimed in the same way,* and as much as possible of the valuable ground in and about the city now occupied as cemeteries be restored to better uses? What if it take us thousands instead of hundreds of years thus to reclaim and elevate such lands, and so practically dispose of our difficulties as to burial for ever?

Anything more puerile and impracticable could surely not be thought of or written by any person who knows the state of our graveyards and cemeteries, and has ever desired their reform. In the "Report on the Practice of Interment in Towns," * (* Clowes and Sons, Stamford Street, 1843.) presented to both Houses of Parliament, it is stated that "there appear to be *no cases in which emanations from human remains in an advanced state of decomposition are not of a deleterious nature*"; and yet Mr. Haden, in the name of progress, seriously proposes to raise and reclaim "*the lowlands of Kent and*

Essex" with decaying human bodies! lie knows that in the course of ages small patches of ground in London and other cities have been raised by piling them with boxes containing bodies, and, accordingly, proceeds to improve the home counties agriculturally in the same wholesome way! Happily our lowlands are not in want of any such "improvement," which is all the more singular as a suggestion from one who poses as a teacher of graveyard reform and aesthetics.

BURYING REPEATEDLY IN THE SAME SOIL.

Official authorities, in opposing urn-burial, have maintained that in "good soil the body may be considered as decomposed and non-existent in from twenty to twenty-five years, and that the same spot may then be used again for the purpose of burying, precisely as if it were virgin soil ". This was in reply to objections as to the great areas of land that must be used for this purpose. "No!" Mr. Holland replies, "the same land can be used at least four times in a century if it is 'good,'- is dry and well drained 'soil' "- a remarkable admission from those who desire to respect or preserve their ancestors' dust! This system of reburying in the same ground again is part of Mr. Haden's pet plan, but what the feeling of the public is about all such plans is shown in the following extract from a lecture by the Rev. Brooke Lambert:

"The results of the improvements in the Tamworth churchyard show me that, however little I may be susceptible to what becomes of my own remains, there is no subject on which people feel more deeply than the disturbance of the remains of their ancestors, and even the displacement of effete memorials of them. From the letters of the better class to the comments of the inhabitants of 'Day's Yard,' who wished that those beneath would come up and punish me and my churchwardens, I find that the prevailing feeling is that the dead ought never to be removed, nor the position of their monuments changed even by a hair's-breadth. *Now whilst our present system of burial remains, such changes in their places of interment must occur.*"

The system of removing the bodies after a lapse of years and burying in the same ground again is carried out in all its ugliness in the Paris cemeteries, but it is so evidently wrong from a sanitary point of view, and also from that of common decency, that it is to be hoped it will never be practised in this country, and it has no chance of success in America, where, more than in any country, the dead receive decent burial. What law, human or divine, justifies this ignoble disturbance of the remains of the dead, and the use of the ground for the burial of other bodies, to be in their turn disinterred in like manner? One may see the effect of it in many exposed bones and skulls in Alpine and North Italian valleys, where thousands of acres of waste land lie around. It is no less offensive, and more dangerous, in large cities; and those who advocate it for our English cemeteries must indeed be at the end of their arguments.

ONE TRUE WAY TO BURIAL REFORM.

There is not, and there never can be, any satisfactory system of disposing of the dead, which does not do, as promptly and as inoffensively as possible, what is now done in the slowest and most horrible manner. Until some better system is devised, cremation is the only method which will rapidly resolve the body into its harmless elements by a process which cannot offend the living, and which shall render the remains of the dead innocuous. This system is also that which gives us the amplest opportunity for making a cemetery beautiful, a blessing instead of a danger to its neighbourhood; by its means we may have memorials preserved from decay; ground from, sacrilege; soil and water from impurity; art not unworthy of its aim; church-burial for all who desire it; space for gardens and groves in our cemeteries; the mindfulness and care of each successive generation; deliverance from the undertaker, and his "effects ; many precious open spaces in cities free from dread or danger; age-enduring cemeteries, in which efforts towards "perpetuating the memory of the dead need not be so delusory as they now are; quiet places, where the ashes of the dead should never be dishonoured, but might find unpolluted rest.

THE MANAGEMENT AND CONTROL OF CEMETERIES.

WHATEVER the future of our cemeteries may be, it is much to be desired that they should not be controlled by trading companies. This is not the way the Americans have established their beautiful cemeteries, which are as well arranged and kept as is possible under the present system of burial. So large and so important a question as the burial of the dead should never be in the hands of those who merely regard it from the point of view of moneymaking. It is well known that the profits from certain cemeteries in some of the pleasantest suburbs of London are very large; the temptation to continue burial in them, longer than decency or sanitary reasons would permit, will probably lead to danger in the future from pollution of air and water. The present state of some of our cemeteries close to London is already dangerous and offensive. On this point Mr. S. Haden makes some just remarks:

"Considering that our reason for discontinuing intra-mural interment was that the soil of the old city graveyards had become so saturated and supersaturated with animal matter that it could no longer properly be called soil, it might have been supposed that, in establishing the new cemeteries, stringent provision would be made that such a pollution of the ground should not again occur; the more so that it must have been foreseen that, by the inevitable extension of the town, the then suburban would become again the intra-mural cemetery, and that the horrors of the old graveyard would thus come to be repeated and multiplied. Not only was no such provision made, but one of the chief of the new companies gave prompt proof of its unfitness to comprehend and to use the powers entrusted to it, by making the extraordinary proposal to bury 1,335,000 bodies in seven acres of ground. Here, since it may not else be believed, is this amazing proposal: 'It has been found,' says the newly installed directors of the General Cemetery Company (Kensal Green), in recommendation of the plans which they are proposing for their future guidance,- 'it has been found that seven acres will contain 133,500 graves; each grave will contain ten coffins; thus, accommodation will be found for 1,335,000 deceased paupers'. The very *naïveté* of this proposal might, one would think, have at once opened the eyes and excited the alarm of those who were conferring on these companies almost unlimited powers, and have prepared them for the abuse of those powers which speedily followed. No such alarm, however, appears to have been excited, and a system of interment founded, we must suppose, on this surprising calculation, was at once Inaugurated and permitted. If, in the old graveyards, the vestries and guardians of the poor saved themselves expense by piling coffin upon coffin till the hole which they had dug would contain no more, the new cemetery companies increased their dividends and propitiated their shareholders by doing precisely the same thing. It is surprising that the Government, which refused to listen to the recommendations of the Board of Health in this matter, should have preferred to entrust the sanitary interests of a great city, and so important a duty as the burial of its dead, to a class of men who, however respectable, had shown themselves ignorant of the very first principles which should govern them in the management of such things.

"Again, apart from the improbability that a mere trading company would prove itself competent to deal with so large, so technical, and so delicate a question as the burial of the dead, it might have been foreseen that the material interests of such a company, its obligations to its shareholders, and its trade associations, could never be in harmony with, but must ever be opposed to, the interests of the public.

The very different spirit with which the new cemeteries in America are undertaken by the leading citizens is well known to many who have travelled there. Cemeteries in America, as well as in Europe, are conducted on various plans. A number of them are under the control of the city authorities, and of course are seldom self-supporting. Others, again, are the property of religious communities, which sometimes manage to pay expenses, and have at times something left for the benefit of the church; but in these cases there is very little security to the owners of burial-places, for the city council or the trustees of the church may at any time pass an ordinance for the removal of the dead to other quarters particularly if the burial-ground be situated in or near a city and has become valuable for other purposes. In that case the last resting-place of the dead is easily condemned as a nuisance, and the consecrated ground is sold for building purposes, for the sake of gain; and in this way, as in our cities, the houses of the living are erected over the graves of the dead.

The plan that has given the greatest satisfaction to the public, and led to the creation of the nobler cemeteries near all the larger cities, and to many beautiful cemeteries in the Western States and in remote places, is that where every lot-holder is a member of the corporation of the cemetery, and where the entire income is devoted to the improvement and perpetual care of the cemetery. Some of these bodies, in addition to forming garden and park-like cemeteries, to which the best in Paris and London are mere stoneyards, have already accumulated a considerable surplus, and there is not the least doubt that in a few years they will have a fund, the interest of which will be more than sufficient to keep the grounds perpetually in complete order.

The following extract is from the Act of Incorporation of the Spring Grove Cemetery at Cincinnati.

"SECTION 6. This Corporation is authorised to purchase, or take by gift or devise, and hold land exempt from execution and from any appropriation to public purposes, for the sole purpose of a cemetery, not exceeding three hundred acres; one hundred and sixty-seven acres of which, such as shall be designated by the directors, shall be exempt from taxation, and the remainder shall be taxed as other lands, untilthe legislature shall otherwise direct. After paying for such land, *all future receipts, whether from the sale 4 of lots, from donations, or otherwise, shall be applied exclusively, under the direction of the board, to laying out, preserving, protecting, and embellishing the cemetery, and the avenues leading thereto, and to paying the necessary expenses of the Corporation.*"

BURIAL : A HORRIBLE PRACTICE

"IF people could see the human body after the process of decomposition sets in, which is as soon as the vital spark ceases to exist, they would not want to be buried; they would be in favour of cremation. If they could go into a dissecting-room and see the horrid sights of the dissecting-table, they would not wish to be buried. Burying the human body, I think, is a horrible thing. If more was known about the human frame while undergoing decomposition, people would turn with horror from the custom of burying their dead. It sometimes takes a human body fifty, sixty, eighty years - yes, longer than that - to decay. Think of it! The remains of a friend lying under six feet of ground, or less, for that length of time, going through the slow stages of decay, and other bodies all this time being buried around these remains. Infants grow up and pass into manhood or womanhood, grow old and get near the door of death; and during all that time the body which was buried in their infancy lies a few feet underground in this sickening state, undergoing the slow process of decay. Think of thousands of such bodies crowded into a few acres of ground, and then reflect that these graves, or many of them, in time fill with water, and that water percolates through the ground and mixes with the springs and wells and rivers from which we drink. Why, if people knew what physicians know, what they have learned in the dissecting-room, they would look upon burning the human body as a beautiful art in comparison with burying it. There is something eminently repulsive to me about the idea of lying a few feet under ground for a century, or perhaps two centuries, going through the process of decomposition. When I die I want my body to be burned. Any unprejudiced mind needs but little time to reflect in forming a conclusion as to which is the better method of disposing of the body. Common sense and reason proclaim in favour of cremation. There is no reason for keeping up the burial custom, but many against it, some of the most practical of which are but too recently developed to need mention. There is nothing repulsive in the idea of cremation. People's prejudice is the only opponent it has. If they could be awakened to a sense of the horror of crowding thousands of. bodies under the ground, to pollute in many instances the air we breathe and the water we drink, their prejudice would be overcome. Cremation would be taken for what it truly is, a beautiful method of disposing of the body." -Dr. S.D. Gross.

PRECAUTIONS AS TO PROOF OF DEATH.

The only serious objection urged from any quarter against the prompt and harmless reduction of the body to its inoffensive parts is that of the supposed immunity it would give to poisoners; and this question is dealt with by Sir Henry Thompson and Mr. Lavel of Paris.

"It has been said, and most naturally, What guarantee is there against poisoning if the remains are burned, and it is no longer possible, as after burial, to reproduce the body for the purpose of examination? It is to my mind a sufficient reply that, regarding only 'the greatest good for the greatest number,' the amount of evil in the shape of disease and death which results from the present system of burial in earth, is infinitely larger than the evil caused by secret poisoning is or could be, even if the practice of the crime were very considerably to increase. Further, the appointment of officers to examine and certify in all cases of death would be an additional and very efficient, safeguard. But-and here I touch on a very important subject-is there reason to believe that our present precautions in the matter of death-certificate against the danger of poisoning are what they ought to be? I think that it must be confessed that they are defective, for not only is our system inadequate to the end proposed, but it is less efficient by comparison than that adopted by foreign governments. Our existing arrangements for ascertaining and registering the cause of death are very lax, and give rise, as we shall see, to serious errors. In order to attain an approach to certitude in this important matter, I contend that it would be most desirable to nominate in every district a properly qualified inspector to certify in all cases to the fact that death has taken place, to satisfy himself as far as possible that no foul play has existed, and to give the certificate accordingly. This would relieve the medical attendant of the deceased from any disagreeable duty relative to inquiry concerning suspicious circumstances, if any have been observed. Such officers exist throughout the large cities of France and Germany, and the system is more or less pursued throughout the provinces. In Paris no burial can take place without the written permission of the *médecin vérificateur*. and whether we adopt cremation or not, such an officer might with advantage be appointed here. It is not generally known that many bodies are buried in this country without any medical certificate at all, and that among these any number of deaths by poison may have taken place for anything that anybody knows. Is it in the provinces chiefly that this lax practice exists? No doubt, and more Particularly in the Principality of Wales. But it occurs also in the heart of London. A good many certificates of death are signed every year in London by some non.. medical persons. In one metropolitan parish, not long ago, which I can name, but do not, above forty deaths were registered in a year on the mere statement of neighbours of the deceased. No medical certificate was procurable, and no inquest was held; the bodies were buried without inquiry. This practice is not illegal, and, in my opinion, it goes far to make a case for the appointment of a *médecin vérificateur*.

"It would be possible, at much less cost than is at present incurred for burial, to preserve, in every case of death, the stomach and a portion of one of the viscera, say for fifteen or twenty years or thereabouts, so that, in the event of any suspicion subsequently occurring, greater facility for examination would exist than by the present method of exhumation. Nothing could be more certain to check the designs of the poisoner than the knowledge that the proofs of his crime, instead of being buried in the earth (from whence, as a fact, not one in a hundred thousand is ever disinterred for examination), are safely preserved in a public office, and that they can be produced against him at any moment. The universal application of this plan, although easily practicable, is, however, obviously unnecessary. It is quite certain that no pretext for such conservation can exist in more than one instance in every five hundred deaths. In the remainder, the fatal result would be attributed without mistake to some natural cause-as decay, fever, consumption, or other malady, the signs of which are clear even to a tyro in the medical art. But in any case in which the slightest doubt arises in the mind of the medical attendant, or in which the precaution is desired or suggested by a relative, or whenever the subject himself may have desired it, nothing would be easier than to make the requisite conservation. As before stated, the existence of an official verificator would relieve the ordinary medical attendant of the case from active interference in the matter. If, then, the public is earnest in its endeavour to render exceedingly difficult or impossible the crime of secret poisoning - and it ought to be so if the objection to cremation on this ground is a valid one - the sooner some measures are taken to this end the better, whether burial in earth or cremation be the future method of treating our dead." -Sir Henry Thompson, in *Contemporary Review.*

"Avant de l'exposer, nous croyons indispensable de répondre a la principale, on pourrait même dire a la seule objection présentée contre la crémation, c'est-a-dire le danger de faire disparaitre les traces d'empoisonnement. M. Cadet a discuté cette question de la manière la plus satisfaisante. Il partage, comme la Commission du Conseil de salubrité, les poisons en deux categories.

"'La premiere, renfermant les poisons qui ne peuvent être retrouvés que dans les cendres: substances organiques, ainsi que le mercure qui est volatil, et le phosphore, ce dernier corps étant en quantité considerable dans notre organisme; La deuxième, comprenant les poisons susceptibles d'être retrouvés: arsenic, antimoine, zinc, cuivre, plomb, etc.; Il est inutile de s'arrêter aux poisons de la premiere catégorie; car tous, excepté le mercure, ne se retrouvent pas plus dans l'inhumation que dans la cremation.'

"M. Cadet examine ensuite la seconde catégorie et prend pour exemple le poison le plus connu, l'arsenic. Il rend compte de nombreuses experiences par lui faites sur des animaux qu'il a empoisonnés par l'arsenic, et qu'il a ensuite incinérés. Il a retrouvé l'arsenic dans les cendres. La société ne serait donc pas désarmée vis-a-vis de tentatives criminelles. M. Cadet ajoute des réflexions extremement justes, qne nous croyons devoir transcrire, parce qu'elles élucident la question de la manière la plus péremptoire.

"'Quand même les poisons ne seraient pas retrouvés dans les cendres, est-ce que cette objection, quoique sérieuse, faite an nom de la médecine légale, que la cremation entrave les investigations de la justice, dans certains cas de crime, est-ce que cette objection, dis-je, pourrait être un obstacle? Elle impose tout simplement la nécessité de prendre des precautions telles, que tout individu tenté de commettre un empoisonnement, ait a réfléchir avant de consommer le crime. Ne peut-on pas établir un mode plus rigoureux de constatation des décès? Une enquête sévère ne pourrait-elle pas être faite avant de délivrer le permis d'incinération d'un cadavre? Un certificat du médecin qui aura donné les soins, constatant la nature de la maladie; un certificat du pharmacien, sur lequel seront transcrites les prescriptions du médecin, pendant la maladie; un certificat du médecin chargé de la verification des décès, indiquant dans quel état il a trouvé le cadavre, avec les signes qui lui sembleraient extraordinaires; le tout envoyé a un médecin contrôleur, seraient des garanties supérieures a celles exigées aujourd'hui pour l'inhumation. En cas de rnort subite ou de mort resultant d'un accident on d'une maladie quelconque, pendant laquelle aucun médecin n'aura été mandé pour donner ses soins, le médecin vérificateur fera une enquête dans la maison du décédé, soit près des parents, soit près des voisins, constatera exactement, dans son certificat, tons les renseignements recueillis, et avisera de suite le médecin contrôleur. Si, dans la visite de ce dernier, ii s'élevait le moindre soupçon, un ordre de s'opposer a la cremation serait envoyé a qui de droit, et le Parquet prévenu du fait. Que pent-on exiger de plus? Toutes les precautions exigées en cas d'empoisonnement ne sont-elles pas suffisantes? Puis, pendant la maladie, ne pourraiton pas exiger du médecin, chaque fois qu'il remarquerait des symptômes douteux ou suspects, qu'il appelat en consultation un on deux confreres, et après examen sérieux, si le doute persistait, qu'il prévint? la justice? Et les matières vomies ne devraient-elles pas être recueillies? Dans de telles circonstances, l'autopsie serait faite ; les viscères, le foie, les organes utiles pour l'analyse chimique, seraient conserves; puis, après un examen attentif de la part du medécin, le corps serait brulé. Il est bien entendu que, sur 1a demande d'un des membres de la famille, ou sur les désirs manifestés par le décédé pendant sa maladie, ou sur les moindres soupcons on indices d'une personne quelconque, l'autopsie aurait lieu de droit.'

"Voilà un ensemble de precautions parfaitement propre a rassurer. La cremation étant autorisée, la police, en vertu des attributions qu'elle possède, et sans qu'il y ait besoin de lois nouvelles, userait de son droit de faire des règlements sur les formalités a remplir. Elle pourrait, dans les cas douteux, prescrire l'autopsie. Mais cette operation laborieuse et dispendieuse ne serait pas la regle generale; car il y a toujours une infinite de cas ou la cause de la rnort est parfaitement connue et ou, par consequent, la cremation ne présente aucun inconvenient. Pour obvier au danger signale par la Commission d'hygiene, d'enlèvement on d'altération des cendres, on pourrait exiger que chaque urne fut scellée et conservée dans le cimetière, pendant plusieurs années; de manière qu'on ne pourrait y porter atteinte sans commettre le delit de violation de sepulture." - *Rapport au Conseil Municipal de Paris,* 1879.

THE STATE OF OUR GREAT SUBURBAN CEMETERIES.

The greater portion of the public probably suppose that the forbidding of burials within the town has saved us from all present danger. The following concerns cemeteries in the immediate suburbs of London-some of those situated in the most pleasant, and which will soon be crowded, suburbs of London.

"During the time that the merits of cremation have been under discussion its advocates might have strengthened their case had they been cognisant of the way in which two of the cemeteries of South London were being managed. We refer to the Battersea Cemetery, controlled by a Burial Board elected by the Vestry of Battersea; and to the Tooting Cemetery, managed by a Burial Board elected by the Vestry of Lambeth. The Tooting Cemetery is not in the parish of Lambeth, but is in the parish of Tooting Graveney, which is comprised within the district of the Wandsworth Board of Works; and the Battersea Cemetery abuts upon the district of the Wandsworth Board. Therefore, the members of the Wandsworth Board are concerned, on behalf of their constituents, in the sanitary condition of both cemeteries. In this matter at least the multiplicity of local authorities has not been without its advantages, for it has required the action of the Wandsworth Board to put a stop to the violation of the Secretary of State's regulations in both cemeteries.

"In April and May an impression prevailed among those resident near the Battersea Cemetery that an exceptional amount of sickness in the neighbourhood, including cases of scarlet fever and diarrhoea, was due to the overcrowded and consequent insanitary condition of the burial-ground. Whatever the cause of the sickness, its existence was a fact. The medical officer of health for West Battersea, Dr. Oakman, reported to the Wandsworth Board that the overcrowding also was a fact, and that it was assuming dangerous and alarming proportions. The Home Office was communicated with, Mr. Holland held an inquiry, and all that had been alleged was proved or admitted. The only person responsible in such a case for the violation of the law is the superintendent of the cemetery, who may be fined for every proved offence. In this instance his resignation was required by the Home Office. He has suffered for the sins of himself and his Board, and has been superseded: and under the management of his successor it is hoped that the regulations of the Secretary of State are being observed.

"A description, in the London weekly organ of the Presbyterians, of a Sunday funeral at Tooting Cemetery, first directed attention to that burial-ground. It was an Irish Catholic funeral, and the mourners lowered the coffin. That was an unusually long one, and, being slightly tilted, it stuck fast half-way down the grave. A gravedigger touched it with his feet, or stood upon it, and some excitement ensued. The object of the writer was to furnish reasons for the discontinuance of Sunday funerals. Incidentally, he mentioned circumstances which pointed to illegalities in the conduct of funerals and to the overcrowding of the ground. The article was read in the Lambeth Vestry. The Burial Board instituted an inquiry into what happened on the Sunday, but ignored the suggested illegalities. They sent a letter to the Vestry declaring the article to be sensational and untrue. The Vestry appointed a committee to inquire into the ignored charges. The Clerk to the Board and the Superintendent of the Cemetery being examined as witnesses made a clean breast of it, and admitted everything. The Vestry Committee reported unanimously that every charge was established.

The irregularities at both the Battersea and the Tooting Cemetery have been of a similar character. In both cases the object was to economise ground and keep down current expenses. The length of time a burial-ground will be available is a mere question of figures if the graves are to be of a certain depth, if there is to be a foot of earth between each coffin, and if no coffin is to be within three or four feet of the top. Dr. Oakman, in his report on the Battersea Cemetery, concludes that, if all regulations are to be carried out, it does not contain sufficient space for a year's burials, and in another part that it must be closed in three years. This contingency it was which led the Board, with ground drained to the depth of eight feet, to permit *graves to be dug deep enough to hold the coffins of fourteen adults or twenty-six children. The percolation of water into these common graves produced decomposition before the graves were filled; and the emanations from them endangered the health of the clergymen and the mourners at each successive funeral up to the fourteenth or the twenty-sixth, as the case might be.* However, as the Board have sacrificed their manager, it may be hoped that these irregularities are things of the past at Battersea.

"With regard to Tooting Cemetery, what the Wandsworth Board did was to appoint Mr. D. C. Noel, medical officer of health for Streatham and Tooting, and Mr. James Barber, the surveyor for the district, to inquire and report. The soil is gravel and clay, the latter predominating; and it therefore retains water. One day, on making a visit, they saw a coffin exposed in a private grave; it had been laid bare at the request of a family for a member of which the grave had been re-opened. The head of the coffin was immersed in one or two inches of black, offensive water. *It was intended to place the next coffin immediately upon that exposed, so that a greater number could be buried in the grave.* Messrs. Noel and Barber addressed a serious of questions to the Lambeth Burial Board, and these were frankly answered. In this case, too, the ground is drained to the depth of eight feet. One question was, 'Is the under-drainage such as to prevent the accumulation of water in graves?' The answer is, 'As far as possible'. Another question was, 'What is the greatest depth to which graves are dug?' The answer is, 'Generally twelve feet, but in some few cases fourteen feet'. Messrs. Noel and Barber infer from these answers that there is no deep under-drainage. The material regulations affecting this cemetery are that there is to be a foot of earth between each coffin, four feet above the top coffin, and no second interment in an earthen grave on the same day unless it be of a member of the same family. The object of the last requirement as it affects common graves is that time may be allowed for the deposit of a foot of earth, which shall be closely rammed down, never to be again disturbed'. It used to be required that graves should be filled up, but the stringency of this regulation was relaxed by the provision that *if a foot of earth were closely rammed down over a coffin, the grave might be available the next day and on each succeeding day until it had received the proper number of coffins to leave the last four feet from the surface.* Messrs. Noel and Barber do not seem to have noticed this.

The questions and answers bearing upon these regulations are as follow: 'Are several coffins buried in one grave on the same day or during the same week?' - 'Yes.' The offence here is in the second interment on the same day; and it was admitted before the Vestry Committee that two interments on the same day were usual, and sometimes there were three. 'Is any layer of earth placed between the coffins in the same common grave, and what thickness?' - '*Hitherto from four inches to six inches, but now one foot.*' 'What is the greatest number of persons over twelve years of age in one common grave?' - 'Up to the present time, six; but now, as a foot of earth is placed between each coffin, only four.' 'What is the greatest number under twelve years of age?' - Ten up to the present time; but, as a foot of earth is to be placed between each coffin, there will only be seven.' It is stated, in answer to one question, that six are the greatest number of coffins buried in a family grave; and the extreme depth of any grave is said, in another answer, to be fourteen feet; whereas, to place one foot of earth between each coffin and to place four feet of earth between the last coffin and the surface of the ground would require that the grave should be originally at least fifteen feet deep, instead of only twelve feet or fourteen feet. Messrs. Noel and Barber find, in conclusion, as the Vestry Committee found before them, that the regulations have been violated; but they have apparently fallen into an error in supposing that this cemetery was subject to the regulation which requires that any and every grave shall be filled up after one interment. They report that the ground is not drained to such a depth and in such effectual manner as shall prevent the accumulation of water in any grave therein, *and that a layer of a foot of earth has not been left over a previously buried coffin.*

"As the municipal government of the Metropolis is under discussion, it may not be inappropriate to point out that, although the Vestry elects the members of a Burial Board, and the Vestry votes the money required by the Board, the Vestry has no control over the Burial Board, the members of which are practically irresponsible. When the Committee of the Lambeth Vestry asked for the attendance of the clerk to the Burial Board and its superintendent at the cemetery, it was found that they were unable to comply with the request without the consent of the Board. The consent was given, but not without a protest against the resolution passed by the Committee, and with the proviso that the permission was not to be treated as a precedent, because the Burial Acts did not authorise the interference of the Vestry in the functions of the Board.

"The enforcement of the law and of the existing regulations will, it is said, necessitate an appeal to the Home Secretary for some relaxations in the case of the metropolitan cemeteries, most of which it is broadly insinuated by the delinquent Boards have been guilty of the same practices. There is something startling in local Boards urging their deliberate breach of well-considered laws as a reason why those laws should be amended. The absorbent properties of soils, the progress of decomposition in different soils, the emanation and diffusion of poisonous gases, the risks of mourners and of adjoining residents, are all elements which have determined the present state of the law, and what is based on scientific fact and experience cannot be changed, to the detriment of the living, for the sake of enabling a local Board to pursue a policy of so-called economy. -*Times*, November 17, 1874.

After reading the foregoing passages in italics no one can say the *fosse commune* of Paris, abominable as it is, is the worst example of the burial of the poor. Do the public, and particularly the women of England, know and acquiesce in the fact that human bodies are stacked, one over the other, with from four inches to a foot of soil between them?

The *Pall Mall Gazette* of the following day contained the following:

"Mr. Holland, the Government Inspector of Burial Grounds, held an official inquiry yesterday into certain allegations which had been made respecting the management of Tooting Cemetery, and the way in which bodies were interred. The most serious charge was that the Cemetery Board had never adopted any measures for the sufficient drainage of the cemetery. A very insufficient system of mere surface drainage was, it had been stated, all that had been provided, and in one case, at least, a coffin had been placed in a grave with water in it sufficient to cover the head of it. This was admitted by the Cemetery

Board, the chairman of which, Mr Robert Taylor, explained that the more efficient drainage of the ground had been under consideration, and that communications had been in progress for the past eight years. Mr. Holland remarked that communication with the main drainage was what was required, and said that unless some steps were speedily taken in the matter the closing of the cemetery would probably be the result. *In the course of the inquiry it was elicited that the entire drainage of the cemetery was conducted into a neighbouring ditch, which discharged itself into the river Wandle, from which many of the inhabitants in its vicinity were accustomed to draw supplies of water."*

After such facts one can sympathise with the declaration of the Rev. Brooke Lambert, in a lecture at Tamworth, that the whole process is, from beginning to end, revolting and disgusting. Such a revolution in our burial arrangements will not come suddenly, but perhaps a little reflection may serve to convince those who have feelings of repulsion to urn-burial, that, as a matter of fact, less dishonour is done to the remains of those whom one loves in subjecting them to a fire which reduces them to ashes which can be carefully preserved, than in allowing them to become the subjects of the loathsome process of corruption first, and then subjecting them to the chance of being ultimately carted away to make room for some metropolitan or local improvement.

Few would not say as much who knew the shocking realities of the cemetery, but those connected with such places do all in their power, for obvious reasons, to keep the painful facts as much concealed as possible from the public. According to the *Times* report, quoted above, a mere incidental allusion in a class paper was what called attention to such a disgraceful and repulsive state of things. And yet we have a Government Inspector of Burials!

A correspondent of *Land and Water*, "E. N. R.", sent to that journal the following:

"How WE BURN OUR DEAD POOR.-Emerging a few days ago from the dismal recesses of a metropolitan railway-station, I chanced to ask my way of an intelligent young fellow who was going in the same direction, and who cheerfully undertook to conduct me. Having, after some consultation, decided the great question of the weather, past, present, and to come, I casually directed his attention to a large cemetery on our right-one of those huge metropolitan burial-grounds established originally far away enough from the haunts of men, but now surrounded by dwellings and closely overlooked by many hundred families.

"To my astonishment I found I had touched a very familiar chord, for my guide, though not himself following the profession, had an intimate connection with the grave-digging interest, his father having 'worked' in that particular cemetery for three-and- twenty years. It was really with the enthusiasm of a man who knows his subject that he imparted to me the inner working life of the Necropolis, first drawing the broad distinction between the 'privates' and the 'commonses,' alluding almost with pathos to the sacred soil devoted to the former, and detailing with professional *sang-froid* the management of the ground dedicated to the latter.

"It is scarcely worth while to reproduce the suburban vernacular in which his remarks were clothed, but he spoke like one who had seen something worth seeing when he exclaimed, 'You should go in there of a night, sometimes, sir, and see them burning the bones and the coffins. You see, they dig up the 'commonses' every twelve years (of course they dare not interfere with the privates), and what they find left of them they burn.'

"The minute particulars of this exhumation and the subsequent cremation were described with a particularity of detail which I am sure I need not attempt; but the moral I draw from this little tale is, that if the poor are to be subjected to cremation at all, surely it would be at least as well to do it in the first instance, and to do it decently, as to postpone the operation for twelve years, and then allow it to be done anyhow!

"To put the matter quite plainly: a corpse buried in 1862 is dug up to-day (in 1874) and burned, very properly; and apart from the miasmatic exhalations of the grave there is an end of it; but admitting that the earth was virgin ground then, it has now been thoroughly tainted, and its disinfecting powers having been largely exhausted, a new corpse, forsooth, is placed in the old grave to tenant it for a new term!

"This is a state of things deserving very serious consideration, for it is clear that it cannot go on without fatal results from a sanitary point of view, for such plans as these are only subterfuges - and, I submit, very improper ones - which serve to shelve the great and pressing question for a time."

EVIDENCE AS TO POLLUTION.

"We," say the reporters of the Sanitary Commission, may safely rest the sanitary part of the case on the single fact, that the placing of the dead body in a grave and covering it with a few feet of earth does not prevent the gases generated by decomposition, together with putrescent matters which they hold in suspension, from penetrating the surrounding soil, and escaping into the air above and the water beneath."

After supporting this statement by illustrations of the enormous force exercised by gases of decomposition, in bursting open leaden coffins whence they issue without restraint, the reporters quote the evidence of Dr. Lyon Playfair to the following effect:

"I have examined," he says, "various churchyards and burial-grounds for the purpose of ascertaining whether the layer of earth above the bodies is sufficient to absorb the putrid gases evolved. The slightest inspection shows that they are not thoroughly absorbed by the soil lying over the bodies. I know several churchyards from which most fetid smells are evolved; and gases with similar odour are emitted from the sides of sewers passing in the vicinity of churchyards, although they may be more than thirty feet from them . . . "

He goes on to estimate the amount of gases which issue from the graveyard, and estimates that for the 52,000 annual interments of the metropolis (a number which has already reached 80,000 in 1873, so rapid is the increase of population. The above was written in 1849), no less a quantity than 2,572,580 cubic feet of gases are emitted, "the whole of which, beyond what is absorbed by the soil, must pass into the water below or the atmosphere above ". The foregoing is but one small item from the long list of illustrative cases proving the fact that no dead body is ever buried within the earth without polluting the soil, the water, and the air around and above it: the extent of the offence produced corresponding with the amount of decaying animal matter subjected to the process.

But "offence" only is proved; is the result not only disagreeable but injurious to the living?

The report referred to gives notable examples of the fatal influence of such effluvia when encountered in a concentrated form; one being that of two grave-diggers who, in 1841, perished in descending into a grave in St. Botolph's Churchyard, Aldgate. Such are, however, extremely exceptional instances; but our reporter goes on to say that there is abundant evidence of the injurious action of these gases in a more diluted state, and cites the well-demonstrated fact that "cholera was unusually prevalent in the immediate neighbourhood of London graveyards ". I cannot cite, on account of its length, a paragraph by Dr. Sutherland, attesting this fact; while the many pages detailing Dr. Milroy's inspection of numerous graveyards are filled with evidence which is quite conclusive, and describes scenes which must be read by those who desire further acquaintance with the subject.

Dr. Waller Lewis reports the mischievous results of breathing the pestiferous air of vaults, and the kind of illness produced by it. His long and elaborate report of the condition of these excavations beneath the churches of the metropolis presents a marvellous view of the phenomena, which, ordinarily hidden in the grave, could be examined here, illustrating the many stages of decay - a condition which he describes as a "disgrace to any 'civilisation.'" But it may be said all this is changed now; intra-mural interment no longer exists; why produce these shocking records of the past?

Precisely because they enable us to know what it is which we have only banished to our suburban cemeteries ; that we may be reminded that the process has not changed; that all this horrible decomposition, removed from our doors - although this will not long be the case, either at Kensal Green or Norwood, to say nothing of some other cemeteries - goes on as ever, and will one day be found in dangerous vicinity to our homes.

STATE OF COUNTRY CHURCHYARDS.

To return to our reporters: we have seen the condition of graveyards in towns, but it will not be undesirable to glance at the evidence relating to the condition of provincial churchyards, where, in the midst of a sparse population, the pure country air circulates with natural freedom - numbers of such spots are mentioned - let one single example be "Cadoxton Churchyard, near Neath ". Respecting this, the reporter writes: "I do not know how otherwise to describe the state of this churchyard than by saying that it is truly and thoroughly abominable. The smell from it is revolting. I could distinctly perceive it in every one of the neighbouring houses which I visited, and in every one of these houses there have been cases of cholera or severe diarrhoea. This is not a selected specimen, some are even worse; for further examples, see the report of Mr. Bowie, describing graveyards at Merthyr-Tydvil, Hawick, Roxburghshire, Greenock, and other places.-Sir H. Thompson.

"At a vestry meeting at East and West Looe, Cornwall, the chairman, the Rev. H. Mayo, Vicar of Talland, described the state of the churchyard at Talland, which is the burial-place for West Looe. Over 8000 bodies had been interred, he said, in a little more than half an acre of ground. The usual depth of graves was about 4½ feet deep, deeper graves being out of the question, owing to the friable nature of the soil, which was being continually turned over. There are no spaces between the graves, and when-ever a person had to be buried the remains of others had of necessity to be disturbed. The sexton had a curious mode of determining whether or not he would be safe in opening any particular spot. He drove a long iron bar down to the requisite depth, and if he met with no substantial obstacle the grave was dug. Only last week, the chairman said he saw a woman beside a newly-opened grave in bitter distress, because the remains of one dear to her had been ruthlessly dug up and exposed. The repeated burials had raised the soil to such an extent that the church appeared to be in a pit, and the polluted atmosphere rendered the sacred edifice unfit for public service. There was constantly oozing from the graves in the higher part of the yard a horrible slime, which came on the floor of the belfry. He was obliged to keep disinfectants for the safety of the ringers. Fresh primroses, which were gathered and placed in the church for decoration on Easter Saturday, were almost black by the following evening, and a scientific friend had told him it was owing to the presence of sulphuretted hydrogen in the atmosphere, in such quantities as would endanger human life. On Ash Wednesday so fetid was the air in the church that the congregation was obliged to withdraw. Under these circumstances it is not surprising that Dr. Holland, the Government Inspector, is of opinion that something must be done to provide a cemetery for the united townships; the ratepayers, however, are determined to put off the evil day of spending money as long as possible, and a motion in favour of taking steps for the formation of a Burial Board was *defeated." -Times,* 1874.

STATE OF FOREIGN CEMETERIES.

"A SPANISH CEMETERY.-There is a little walled- in spot of sandy, rocky ground, some two miles outside the town from which I write - it is the cimenterio, where at last the bones of the Spanish peasant are laid in peace, waiting for the touch of that magic wand which one day is to make all things new. I entered that sacred ground a few nights since for the first time. Much as I had heard of the beauty of burial-yards abroad, I looked at least for decency and cleanliness. The first thing that struck me as I opened the gate and took off my hat was the sickly, putrid smell, that well-nigh caused me to vomit. Close before me, on a rough hewn and unlettered stone, stood two tiny coffins; the lids (always of glass) were not screwed down. I pushed one aside, and there, beautiful even in death, were the rich tresses and pink cheeks of a child of some eight summers. The other was the coffin of an infant. Both bodies were wrapped, as is customary here, in coloured silver paper-for the clothes are *burnt* invariably, as they might be a temptation to some dishonest person to exhume the coffin from its shallow grave. Just then I looked down, and lo! the whole place was covered with human bones, lying on the surface. The evening breeze rose and fell; coming from the distant Sierra Morena, and wafted to my feet - it *clung around* my feet - a light loose mass of long and tangled hair. Stooping down to look, I saw that there was plenty of it about; on the gravestones, and around the dry thistles, which grew in abundance, it twined and clung. There was no grass, no turf-only sand, and rocks peeping out. This, then, was the end of life's brief drama here: the rude end of a still ruder life! I saw no tombstones worthy of the name. I asked the old grave-digger when would he bury the two little coffins? 'Manana' (to-morrow), he answered; but the place is so full, I hardly know where to scrape a hole.' "- *Macmillan's Magazine.*

Similar unpleasant scenes may be witnessed in many of the fairest mountain districts of Europe, where, notwithstanding thousands of acres of Italy and Switzerland lying waste around, the bones are dug up and exposed for no other "reason" than "want of room"!

THE CEMETERIES OF PARIS.

This nuisance, in various ways bound up with superstition, is unseen in France, but, to anyone accustomed to associate cemeteries with gardens more or less beautiful, the cemeteries of Paris are far from being agreeable. In these, human love does not fail in its testimony; but such are the evils of overcrowding, of still following plans less evidently wrong when the city was much smaller, and of the odious system of using the same ground for interments many times over, that the best aspects of these cemeteries are painful. Nothing more agreeable is to be seen than crowded stones, and whole acres covered with decaying blackened "immortelles ". In the portions devoted to the graves of the rich, or of such as passed on their way to the grave by the paths of fame or glory, a little chapel or a ponderous tomb often prevents for a time the dust of individuals from mingling with the common clay of their neighbours, and the earth is not used merely as a deodorising medium, as in other parts of the same cemetery.

Where the poorer people bury their dead in this part of the graveyard may be seen a most revolting mode of sepulture. A very wide trench or *fosse* is cut, broad enough to hold two rows of coffins placed across it, and one hundred yards or so in length. Here they are rapidly stowed in one after another, close together, no earth between the coffins, and wherever the coffins, which are very fragile, happen to be short, so that a little space is left between the two rows, those of children are placed in lengthwise between them to economise space; the whole being done much as a workman would pack bricks together. This is the *fosse commune,* or grave of the humble class of people, who cannot afford to pay for the ground. The remains of these people thus dishonoured are not even allowed to rest in the grave, such as it is, but after the lapse of a short time their bones are dug up and the ground prepared for another "crop". A cutting, 13 to 14 feet wide, with the earth thrown up in high banks on either side, a priest standing at one part near a slope formed by the slight covering thrown over the buried of that day, and, frequently, a little crowd of mourners and friends, bearing a coffin.

They hand it to the man in the bottom of the trench, who packs it beside the others without placing a particle of earth between; the priest says a few words, and sprinkles a few drops of water on the coffin and clay; some of the mourners weep, but are soon moved out by another little crowd, with its dead, and so on till the long and wide trench is full. They do not even take the trouble to throw a little earth against the coffins last put in, but simply place a rough board against them for the night. Those places not paid for in perpetuity are completely cleared out, dug up, and used again after a few years. The wooden crosses, little headstones, and countless ornaments are carted away or are thrown together in great heaps, the crosses and consumable parts being generally sent to the hospitals as fuel. The headstones from such a clearance (when not claimed in good time by their owners) go to make the drainage of a drive, or for some similar end. And yet these people, who cannot afford to pay for the ground in perpetuity, go on erecting inscribed headstones, and bringing often their little tokens of love, knowing well that a few years will sweep away these, and that afterwards they cannot even tell where is the dust of those that have been taken from them. One day, when in the Cemetery of Mont Parnasse, I saw the workmen making a new road, the bottom of which was formed of broken headstones, many of them bearing a date four years before. These had been placed on ground that had not been paid for in perpetuity, and were consequently grubbed up at the end of a few years when the ground was required again for another series of these disgusting interments. The plan is, however, on the whole, more decent and less dangerous than the London one of piling many bodies one over the other, with a very little soil between each.

DISRESPECT AND INSULT TO THE DEAD.

A correspondent of the *Medical Times and Gazette,* writing from Bordeaux, says:

" . . . The earth around one of the oldest churches in Bordeaux seems to have something peculiarly antiseptic in its nature, so that the bodies buried during ages were converted into mummies. During some alterations at the beginning of this century these bodies were laid bare, and instead of being decently buried again, they were taken out of their resting-places and ranged upright, in a row, around a crypt under the bell-tower of the church of St. Michel. Here they constitute a disgusting and demoralising show, which is visited by crowds of people, and I am afraid that the clergy of the church are not ashamed to pocket the profits. A rough fellow, with a candle on the end of a stick, such as they have in wine- cellars, goes round as showman. He taps and thumps the bodies to show that they are perfectly sound, tough like leather trunks, and not the least brittle. 'See here, gentlemen, is a very tall man; see how powerful his muscles must have been, and what excellent calves he has now! The next is the body of a young woman. Remark the excellent preservation of her chemise, though it was buried 400 years ago; and see! it is trimmed with lace! The next, gentlemen, is a priest; you can see his *soutane* with the buttons on it. There is a woman with a dreadful chasm in her breast; she had a cancer. The next four are a family poisoned with mushrooms; observe the contortions on their faces from the *coliques* they suffered. See next a very old man with his wig still awry upon his pate. The next is a poor *miserable* that was buried alive. See how his head is turned to one side and the body half turned round, in the frantic effort to get out of the coffin, with his mouth open and gasping.' (It is quiet true that the attitude is singular, but it does not warrant the inference which the showman draws from it.) But enough of this disgusting mercenary exhibition of the human body in its lowest state of humiliation. If the guardians of consecrated sepulchres, in which people have paid an honest fee to be buried, are to dig them up and cart them off as in England, or make a show of them as here, why I can only say that 'cremation' will gain a good many converts. Anyone would prefer urn-burial to the chance of being thus made a spectacle. So good, too, it must be for the rising population, to take off the edge of any salutary horror they may feel at death and decay, or of reverence for the dead!

"MALTA.-One of the chief sights of Malta is the crypt of the Franciscan Convent, in which are preserved the dried bodies of the monks. A monk, holding a lighted candle, went down before us into the vault or crypt, into which air and a small allowance of daylight are admitted by windows placed high up in the roof. All round the crypt, in niches, stood the bodies of former tenants of the convent, and a most ghastly sight they were. Each figure was dressed in a monk's habit and cowl, and was propped up by a wooden bar placed before the waist. Our guide held the light close to each figure, so that we might be able to see all the revolting details. In one niche the still corpulent figure of a monk lolled against the wooden bar which supported him: the jaw had sunk, and the tongue hung out of the mouth. In another a tall figure stood with its withered hands, like mouldy parchment, crossed in front of it; the brown beard still clung to the chin, but the eyes had decayed away, and the lips had shrunk back from the teeth, giving the face a dreadful leering expression, greatly at variance with the reverent attitude of the hands. The sight of these horrible figures made me a stronger believer than ever in the advisability of burning the dead. I fancy even the prejudice with which public opinion clings to the unhealthy and disgusting plan of endeavouring to preserve the bodies of the dead would receive a slight shake on having ocular demonstration of what very horrible things our mortal remains must become, even under the most favourable circumstances. The old heathen did very wisely in destroying, as far as possible, all disgusting associations with death; and surely there is much less shock to sentiment in having the ashes of those we have 'loved and lost' carefully guarded in a cinerary urn, than knowing that the body is lying festering below, amid all the noxious abominations of churchyard earth." -Edith Osborn, *Twelve Months in Southern Europe.*

A correspondent of the *Times* writes from Alexandria:

Cremation and Urn-Burial; or, The Cemeteries of the Future

"The other day, at Sakhara, I saw nine camels pacing down from the mummy pits to the bank of the river, laden with nets, in which were femora, tibia, and other bony bits of the human form, some two hundredweight in each net, on each side of the camel. Among the pits there were people busily engaged in searching out, sifting and sorting the bones which almost crust the ground. On inquiry I learned that the cargoes with which the camels were laden would be sent down to Alexandria, and thence be shipped to English manure manufacturers. They make excellent manure, I am told, particularly for Swedes and other turnips. The trade is brisk, and has been going on for years, and may go on for many more. It is a strange fate-to preserve one's skeleton for thousands of years in order that there may be fine Southdowns and Cheviots in a distant land!"

"ENGLISH VAULTS.-When it is necessary, as sometimes it must be, to disturb interments not older than the rest, but of a more ambitious character, the spectacles disclosed are such as to make one envy the pauper, his quicker return to Dame Nature's all-teeming, all-receiving bosom. The family vaults of old parish churches are, as anybody may know, the scene of more grotesque incidents, more sacrilegious robberies, more horrible profaneness, than any spots above ground, however open to the every-day world. Nuisances, as they certainly are, they suffer a Nemesis in the dishonour and contempt they often bring on the poor remains they were designed to protect and *honour*." -*Times,* Leading Article, 1874.

FUNERAL CEREMONY.

"Our whole process of sepulture, with its wood and lead coffins (only necessitated by our custom of keeping the dead so long in our houses) and brick vaults, seems to me almost like an insult to God and a defiance of Nature's laws, endeavouring as we do - how vainly! - to impede or even prevent the carrying out of those laws.

"And now, sir, one word on a subject akin to the above, not necessarily combined with it as regards reform, though in my opinion they should go hand in hand. I allude to the processes and operations to which, dead and alive, we have to submit from the moment of death to that of placing the remains in the grave. how long, I would ask, are we to be subjected to the tyranny of custom and undertakers? How long are we to be smothered with flowing hatbands, scarves, and mourning cloaks, mobbed and overpowered by mutes, ostrich feathers, &c.? How long are we to continue to see the remains of some quiet old gentleman or lady, who perhaps never in his or her life sat behind anything more exalted than a small pony, drawn to their last home by four long-tailed black horses, or some one who, having lived unloved, dies unmourned, and is yet attended to his grave by half a dozen hired mourners at 5s. per day and their beer? Truly, it is all vanity and vexation of spirit - a mere mockery of woe; a prolongation and refining of misery to the really miserable, a source of ridicule and contempt to those who are actors or spectators; costly to all, far, far beyond its value; and ruinous to many; hateful, and an abomination to all; yet submitted to by all, because none have the moral courage to speak against it and act in defiance of it.

"LORD ESSEX."

CREMATION, NATURE'S PROCESS.

"It is easily demonstrable that cremation is Nature's one only process of resolving lifeless matter into its elements, and that under any circumstances it is but a question whether this mode of consuming the lifeless human body shall occupy a longer or a shorter period. The sun is the source of all chemical change. All chemical action is, in fact, a form of cremation. Life itself is carried on by a process of combustion, and all human beings are carrying on the process within them from the cradle to the grave. When the fire which effects this result is extinguished, we should get rid of the body by Nature's most rapid means of cremation and burn it. Nature gets rid of fermenting, corrupting matter by this means, and often indicates the consummation she is aiming at by spontaneous combustion.

"If inhumation had been Nature's best process of getting rid of dead animal and vegetable matter, we may depend upon it that the beasts would have instinctively buried their dead. But not only has she not implanted such an instinct, but she has developed birds and savage beasts to feed on garbage and carrion, and by this means to cremate what would otherwise prove noxious and pestilential, by the process of digestion. Fire was always considered to be a sacred element by the ancients. It was never allowed to expire in the temples, and it still burns as an emblem of purity and intelligence before the altar. Cremation was esteemed the acceptable mode of making an offering. 'I will *purge* with fire,' 'I will not suffer My Holy One to see *corruption*,' are familiar texts. Which, then, is the greater desecration of human remains, to burn them with fire or to give them over to the earth and to a long process of slow combustion and corruption-a corruption that one instinctively revolts at, and which is too horrible to be contemplated?

"Cremation ensures the purity of the atmosphere and of the springs, both of which are contaminated to a frightful and incalculable extent by the present system of interment, as we shall immediately show. Data shall be given which will put the state of things resulting from this system in its most appalling light. The registered deaths in the

United Kingdom for 1874 were 699,747. Taking this as an approximate annual death registry for Great Britain, and allowing ten years for the complete resolution of the body under the present mode of interment - a period, it is believed, considerably below the mark - we have in the kingdom nearly seven millions of dead bodies lying in various stages of decomposition, and giving off noxious exhalations by means of percolation to the atmosphere, and by sending down contaminating matter to the subterranean -reservoirs. Calculating for London alone, there were, in 1872, 76,634 deaths; there are therefore, at a rough estimate, nearly a million of human bodies festering in its immediate neighbourhood. Fortunately for the springs, some of the cemeteries are on clayey soils, and bodies interred in them are to a certain extent locked up in their clay vaults, only to be a source of mischief when they are opened. Some of these graves have been described, by one who is bound to know, as 'very cesspools' of human remains, which give forth their noxious gases whenever broken into for the purpose of some fresh interment, as many a mourner has experienced to his cost. Bodies, on the other hand, which have been buried in sandy soils are more quickly resolved, say in some six or seven years. Interments in sandy soils, however, are more likely to endanger the health of the living, for by percolation the fluids contaminate the springs and the foul gases are exhaled into the atmosphere. If human remains were buried in quick lime their dissolution would be more rapidly effected; but on the slightest reflection it is perceived that this method is but a method of cremation. Why not, therefore, at once adopt the more direct, complete, and rapid progress of cremation, and ensure the purity of the air and water for the benefit of the living? Deference should be paid to custom and to prejudice. We would not interfere with the sanctity of the funeral rite, nor deprive the Church of its dues. It would be a good bargain if we could obtain the adoption of cremation at the price of double fees. It is quite possible to have cremation with precisely the same funeral ceremonies as at present."
-W. CAVE THOMAS, *Social Notes*.

REASONS AGAINST COFFINLESS BURIAL, OR THE "EARTH TO EARTH" SYSTEM.

"Though strongly averse to half measures on a question of such vital and universal importance, I hail with pleasure Mr. Seymour Haden's proposals concerning reform in the undertaker department as a step in the right direction, but still am inclined to go deeper and dive to the root of the evil, by maintaining the importance of a more decided change.

"In the first place, I would remark that one great argument in favour of cremation is that the present poisoning of our watercourses and springs would be for ever at an end so far as our cemeteries arc concerned, but that if Mr. Seymour Haden's proposals should be adopted (admirable in intention as they are), still the evil would remain, and not only remain, but be aggravated doubly-ay, trebly.

"To illustrate my meaning, suppose a cemetery in which there are, say, for the sake of argument, thirty interments weekly. Under the present system, which is opposed to Nature, and revolting in the extreme, the thirty bodies encased in the strong leaden or oaken prisons decompose slowly, taking years over that operation, and do not con-taminate the surrounding earth or springs or vitiate the air in at all a sudden manner.

"But turn now to the other picture; look at it in the new light, and suppose - horrible supposition! - that the thirty bodies (in which the process of decomposition has already set in while above ground), encased in some light covering, as wickerwork for instance, about as durable when compared with lead or oak as paper is to sackcloth, are fast mingling with that powerful earth, and as speedily carrying poison to our springs and along our watercourses. A change is needed, and a change is demanded, but Heaven defend us from our friends,' if we are to supply the present slow contamination of our springs by one doubly more speedy and efficacious.

"Secondly, by resolving all that was mortal of one we loved into our mother earth, by means of interment in slender cases instead of leaden or oaken coffins, we effect that operation in a far speedier manner, though with the necessary delay of some years. But what need is there of any delay? Why retard Nature instead of rapidly furthering her ends? I appeal to the gentler sex, whose attention has now been drawn to this vital yet depressing subject, and ask them whether, for mock sentiment's sake, the fair human body should slowly and for years go through that dreadful process, when in an hour or two, at the expense of no real sentiment (I use the expression in its loftiest and genuine sense), all that Nature demands is accomplished?

"'I presume no one is likely to question Mr. Seymour Haden's contention that a dead body is more quickly and innocuously resolved into its elements and assimilated, in proportion as it is brought in closer proximity with the earth. This is common knowledge. What I had hoped to see stated was how far a process of burial without coffins is likely to be less injurious to the community. Will not noxious gases still arise, and would, not water be polluted by percolation from a burial-ground? This seems the real question at issue. Before the body has decayed and been assimilated, is its condition not likely to be as injurious, or nearly so, as under the present system? In every burial-ground there would be dead bodies constantly brought in, and therefore decay would be constantly going on. I do not yet see how, unless people stop dying, the mere quickening of the decay will do away with all evil results, though it may modify their harmfulness. What I understand the advocates of cremation to argue is that under their system all poisonous influence would be avoided. Mr. Seymour Haden urges as a result of his system that the same ground might be used over and over again at frequent intervals. To my mind it would be more painful to dig up and destroy the graves of those we loved, than to preserve only their ashes.'- 'Y' in *Times*.

"The question is, will the abolition of coffins always improve matters? The interment of the body in a mere shroud is no new idea, and under many a lych-gate in our old churchyards have such uncoffined corpses been borne. Indeed it has not died out yet. In county Kildare there resides an ancient family, the deceased members of which are always carried to the graveyard at Tully in this manner. It is considered in the neighbourhood to be an eccentric practice, but, nevertheless, the family observe this peculiarity, and have done so from time immemorial. There can be no doubt that in ancient times the practice was almost universal amongst those who buried their dead. It is hoped that by dispensing with the coffin the body will sooner return to the elements, about which there can be no question, provided that the earth in which it is interred be a suitable one. But that is not always the case, for under certain circumstances of humidity in the soil the muscular fibres of the body are, for instance, converted into adipocere, and this substance has been even sought for to use as cart-grease. Soils which keep out the atmospheric air are nearly always favourable to the generation of this substance. Here it need hardly be stated the earth is unsuitable for sepultural purposes. The ground chosen for a cemetery may not only be too damp and clayey, and impervious to air and moisture, but it may be of too open a character. Were we to bury in light gravelly soil of this class without coffins, it is not unlikely that the foul gases would levitate faster than they ought to do. From graves with plural interments the danger would be increased. We do not know exactly why coffins were originally resorted to, but it is just possible that our forefathers discovered that in certain soils the earlier and fouler stages of decomposition proceeded at too rapid a pace for the comfort of the living. The depurative power of the soil was not equal to the strain cast upon it.

"This is not an altogether theoretical statement, for an eminent foreigner has noticed that this is the case in graveyards which he had visited. A coffin may, therefore, be a desirable thing under some circumstances. It is a fit question to consider also whether it would be safe to bury the body of a man who perished (for instance) from smallpox without protecting it by a coffin. Mischief would be less likely to result after such a lapse of time as was found necessary to destroy the coffin. Here it is where the advantages of cremation appear, for with the body is burned up all disease germs whatsoever. The thing to consider is, how many persons die from contagious diseases the germs of which not even the earth can destroy? It is not so much a question of coffin or no coffin. When the Minchinhampton churchyard was disturbed, and the black earth carted to the gardens round about, the population was simply decimated; and the same would have occurred, one would imagine, even if the coffin earth had been absent.' -*Sanitary Record.*

"As a man of science, we think Mr. Haden has committed the very pardonable error of trying to claim too much for his method; and the confiding reader of the first part of his letter would be led to infer that organic matter is not only incapable of putrefaction, in the ordinary sense, if buried in the earth, but that it is incapable of working any harm. The ordinary reader could infer nothing else from the following paragraph, for instance, in which the high authority of Mr. Simon is invoked by Mr. Haden:

"'Nor, again, is the effect of the earth upon fluids in a state of putrescence at all less remarkable than upon solids, filtration through a few feet of common earth being sufficient to deprive the foulest water of any amount of animal or other putrid matter contained in it. We need go no further for a proof of this than to a certain pump in Bishopsgate Street which stands opposite the rails of the old churchyard there, and of which Mr. Simon, the distinguished medical officer of the Privy Council, gives us the following interesting account: "The water from this well is perfectly bright, clear, and even brilliant; it has an agreeable soft taste, and is much esteemed by the inhabitants of the parish, though, as will be seen by the subjoined analysis, it is an exceedingly hard water . . . (yielding carbonates of lime and magnesia, sulphate of lime, chloride of sodium, nitrates of potash, soda, magnesia, and ammonia, silica, and phosphate of lime, but of organic matter none or scarcely a trace). . . . The quantity of nitrates in this water is very remarkable. These salts are doubtless derived from the decomposition of animal matter in the adjacent churchyard. Their presence, conjoined with the inconsiderable quantity of organic matter which the water contains, illustrates in a very forcible manner the power that the earth possesses of depriving the water that percolates it of any animal matter it may hold in solution; and, moreover, shows in how complete and rapid a manner the process is effected. In this case the distance of the well from the churchyard is little more than the breadth of the footpath, and yet this short extent of intervening ground has, by virtue of the oxidising power of the earth, been sufficient wholly to decompose and render inoffensive the liquid animal matter that has oozed from the putrefying corpses in the churchyard.'"

"The above, we are afraid, would be likely to cause a false impression, for it is a well-ascertained fact that the surest carrier and most fruitful nidus of zymotic contagion is this brilliant, enticing-looking water, charged with the nitrates which result from organic decomposition.

"What, for example, was the history of the Broad Street pump which proved so fatal during the cholera epidemic of 1854? Was its water foul, thick, and stinking? Unfortunately not. It was the purest-looking and most enticing water to be found in the neighbourhood, and people came from a distance to get it. Yet there can be no doubt that it carried cholera to many who drank it; and its analysis showed that in composition it was very similar to the water near the graveyard in Bishopsgate Street alluded to by Mr. Haden. We are afraid Mr. Haden will have to confess that at present the only known method of making organic matter certainly harmless is the process of cremation." - *The Lancet.*

Speaking of the soil, Mr. Haden says:

"It is the most potent antiseptic known. . . . It is resolvent and re-formative as well; what under the influence of the air was putrefaction, in the earth is resolution; what was offensive becomes inoffensive; what was decay, a process of transmutation. Now the word 'antiseptic' means that which opposes putrefaction. But it is not true either that the soil is the most potent antiseptic known, or, in a strict sense, that it is antiseptic at all. When a body is buried naked in the soil it putrefies, and its organic components are resolved, for the most part, into gaseous substances. Some of those substances are exceedingly fetid, just as they are when, under ordinary atmospheric conditions, they are evolved from a body putrefying above ground. When, however, the gases are made to traverse a layer of soil several feet in depth, the fetid portion of them is oxidised by the atmospheric oxygen contained in the soil, and so converted into inodorous matter, such, for example, as carbolic acid, or, what is equivalent, it is slowly burnt. Combination with oxygen is promoted by the mechanical action of porous substances like soil. Again, every drop of rain water falling upon the ground and percolating the soil contains oxygen, which in that state of solution exerts a strong oxidising action. If it were true that the soil is even a potent antiseptic in the accepted sense of the word, then it would follow that the burial of a body naked in the soil would favour its preservation. But this is exactly what Mr. Haden does not desire, though it is certainly what would result from the substitution of wickerwork coffins for those of wood, if the soil were an antiseptic. If I correctly interpret Mr. Haden's letter, one reason for his objecting to the use of ordinary coffins is that what he calls the pro-cess of transmutation - an improper application of the word when applied to such changes as he refers to- is retarded. Now, if this be the case, the evolution of gases from a body enclosed in an ordinary coffin will continue for a much longer time than from a body buried naked in the soil; and, therefore, their oxidation in the former is, *pro tanto*, more likely to be complete than in the latter." - "X" in *Times*.

THE BISHOP OF MANCHESTER ON THE EVILS AND WASTE OF BURIAL, AND ON CREMATION.

THE remarks of the Right Rev, the Lord Bishop of Manchester, made during the opening of the Social Science Congress at Manchester, October 1, 1879, are worthy of being reproduced here. He said:

"I now draw attention to the provision made in our cities for interment of the dead. On Friday last I consecrated a portion of a new cemetery, provided by the Corporation on the south side cf Manchester, fully five miles from the centre of the city, containing ninety-seven acres, at a cost, including the land, the fencing, the laying out, and the inevitable three or four chapels, of £100,000. It is very beautiful; but two thoughts occurred to me as I was consecrating the portion of it assigned to those who desire to be buried according to the rites of the Church of England. In the first place, this is a long distance for the poor to bring their dead; in the second place, here is another hundred acres of land withdrawn from the food-producing area of the country for ever. I do not think we always observe or calculate how much this area is being gradually contracted by the infinite number of works and processes, requiring space, but not producing food, which are encroaching upon it more and more every year; nor to what extent the power of the country to support its population is reduced thereby. *Jam pauca aratro jugera regioe Moles relinquent.'* In times of peace and plenty we can afford to be indifferent to this consideration; but I can easily conceive the existence of circumstances which would make this a very serious condition indeed. I feel convinced that before long we shall have to face this problem, ' How to bury our dead out of our sight,' more practically and more seriously than we have hitherto done. In the same sense in which the' Sabbath was made for man, not man for the Sabbath,' I hold that the earth was made not for the dead, but for the living. *No intelligent faith can suppose that any Christian doctrine is affectcd by the manner in which, or the time in which, this mortal body of ours crumbles into dust and sees corruption.* I admit that my instincts and sentiments - the result, however, probably of association more than of anything else - are somewhat revolted by the idea of cremation. But they are perhaps illogical and unreasonable sentiments. Sir Henry Thompson has stated the case in a calm and thoughtful paper, which shows how little ground there is for the somewhat morbid sentiments that indeed prevail in relation to the whole subject of the interment of the dead. All I call attention to is that it is a subject that will have to be seriously considered before long. Cemeteries are becoming not only a difficulty, an expense, and an inconvenience, but an actual danger."

TURKISH CEMETERIES.

The following has been sent me, since the passing of the foregoing pages through the press, by Mr. C. W. Quin, who recently lived some years at Constantinople:

"It is a generally accepted but erroneous notion that the Turks take especial pains to keep the graves of their dead free from desecration. Turkish cemeteries are simply picturesque cypress woods in all their natural wildness, not the slightest effort being made either to cultivate or even level them. They are generally unenclosed, except when they are attached to mosques, or are surrounded by houses, as in the case of the cemetery of the Dancing Dervishes in Pera, where the famous French renegade, Ahmed Pasha, the Comte de Bonneval, is buried. There are two large cemeteries in Pera, known respectively as the Grand and the Petit Champs des Morts. They are both being gradually eaten up by the encroachments of the builders and the public. It is a painful sight for a European to see human bones protruding from graves which have been scratched up by the numberless herds of wild dogs. The Turks bury their bodies without coffins; a single parish coffin, so to speak, being used to convey the body to the grave. The body is placed in the earth in its ' habit as it lived'. The Turkish mode of burial is about the most contrary to sanitary rules that could have been devised. The graves are very shallow, sometimes not more than a foot in depth, the reason for this being that most old-fashioned Turks still retain the superstition that the soul does not leave the body until some time after burial, when it is drawn from the grave by the Angel of Death, who would find great difficulty in performing his task if the body was buried too deeply. The consequence of this is, that in warm weather a horrible stench arises from the cemeteries. The walk from the Golden Horn to the Sea of Marmora, outside the famous Byzantine land walls, is replete with historical associations at every step of the seven miles; but it can only be taken with comfort in cool weather, the stench from the great cemetery outside the Adrianople Gate being too great to be borne. Frightful incidents are told of dogs and wolves rifling the graves of the dead; and during the severe winter of 1874-75 two

73

wolves were found in the English cemetery at Pancaldi, outside Pera, scratching at the newly made grave of a respected member of the English colony. They had already scratched their way down to the coffin."

DESECRATION OF THE WHITFIELD BURIAL-GROUND.

Here is an instance, reported in the daily papers during the last few weeks, of the fate of burial- grounds in London:

"Nathan Woolfe Jacobson, of 311 and 312 Oxford Street, was on Wednesday summoned by William Rouch, inspector of nuisances for the parish of St. Pancras, for having on 30th March removed the remains of human bodies from a portion of a disused burial-ground on the north side of the Congregational Chapel, formerly George Whitfield's Tabernacle, in Tottenham Court Road, without a licence, contrary to the provisions of the Burials Acts. These proceedings were instituted by the Vestry in the interests of the public health as well as of public decency. The Rev. George Whitfield in 1756 founded a chapel or tabernacle, with a piece of ground of about half an acre attached to it as a burying-ground, and held the land upon lease. The ground was not consecrated. The lease expired in 1827, and then the ground was closed for some three years. In 1831, however, the trustees of the chapel purchased the copyhold, but, in order to secure the money borrowed, they mortgaged the land to a Mr. Tudor, who ultimately foreclosed, and in 1862, the land being sold by order of the Court of Chancery, the defendant became the purchaser of two-thirds of it. Now, the first interment in the ground had taken place on November 19, 1756, and the last in October, 1853. The ground was used for ninety-seven years as a place of interment, and 30,000 bodies were interred in the half-acre of ground during that time. The defendant appeared to have purchased it with a view to some building speculation, and in 1863 he began to move some of the bodies from one part of the ground to the other. He was immediately summoned to that court, and fined by Mr. Knox £5 and costs. He then desisted, and allowed the ground to become the receptacle of refuse, until it became such a nuisance that the sanitary authorities proceeded to fence it in with the view of making ornamental grounds. Thereupon the defendant filed a bill in Chancery, and in February, 1883, succeeded in obtaining a decree, restraining them from interference. Having obtained that decree in his favour, he had now resumed his attempt to excavate the ground and to disturb the remains of the dead. He thought the magistrate, after hearing the evidence, would consider the defendant's proceedings to be most in decent, and to call for his intervention.

"Mr. William Rouch, inspector of nuisances, said he knew Whitfield's burial-ground, the area of which is about half an acre. He had known, it thirty years. It had been closed about 1853. It was thickly studded with graves in every part, and was in a populous neighbourhood. On Tuesday he went to the ground, which was then enclosed by a high hoarding. He was refused admission, but subsequently was admitted by an order from the magistrate. He found men at work excavating the ground, and there were horses and carts being loaded. Men were digging, and earth and human bones were being dug out together. He saw parts of human skulls, rib bones, leg bones, shoulder bones, &c. There were decayed pieces of wood, which had formed parts of coffins. There were about a bushel of human bones in a box near the carts which were being loaded, and in a trench he found about a cart- load of human bones, which had been previously dug out; there was only a sprinkling of earth over them. The workmen said they had no appointed shoot for the mould, and that they took it to Ilaverstock Hill or elsewhere. He had visited the place again on Wednesday and found the men still at work. Four horses and carts were being loaded, and the mould taken away through the streets.

"Mr. Harston argued that the burial-place not being consecrated it did not come within the Act, as there had been no interments there since 1853, and the Act was not passed till 1857. It had been so decided by the Court of Queen's Bench in the case of *Foster and Dodd,* and when this matter was re- cently before the Master of the Rolls. he said there was nothing whatever to prevent the defendant building on it. The point had been fought out over and over again, and had always ended in one way. I can assure you we do not wish to make any scandal. Mr. Newton - ' But it is a scandal'. Mr. Harston- ' You must remember the Bank of England is built on an ancient burying-ground'. Mr. Newton-' I know nothing of that. Still it is a scandal that this thing should be permitted.'"

VIOLATION OF THE GRAVES AT ST. DENIS.

The other day I came across a somewhat rare little *brochure* - an account of the violation of the royal sepulchres of St. Denis during the first French Revolution:

"The work of destruction and sacrilege commenced early in October, 1793, and lasted all the month. The first corpse found was that of Henri IV., the once beloved Henri de Navarre. Some curiosity, if not affection, still seems to have lingered even among those patriots who had constituted themselves body-snatchers, and the Bearnais was propped up against the church wall in his shroud, and became quite an attraction for the crowd. One of the Republican Guards even condescended to cut off the king's grey, upturned moustache, and place it on his lip; another removed the beard, which he declared he would keep as a relic. After these marks of attention were exhausted, the body was thrown into a huge pit filled with quicklime, into which successively followed those of its ancestors and descendants.

"On the next day the corpses of Henri IV.'s wife, Marie de Medicis, that of his son, Louis XIII., and that of his grandson, Louis XIV., were added to this. The body of the Sun King (as Louis XIV.'s courtiers loved to call him) was as ' black as ink'. What a contrast to that majestic, bewigged head, as we see it on the canvas of Le Brun and Rigault, must not that poor blackened skull have been! The body of the Grand Monarch's wife and that of his son the Dauphin (father of Louis XV.) followed. All these, and especially the latter, were in a state of shocking decay.

"The following day poor harmless Marie Leczinska's body was torn from its resting-place, as also were those of the Grand Dauphin,' the Duke of Burgundy and his wife, and several other princes and princesses of the same race, including three daughters of Louis XV. All these were in a state of terrible decomposition, and in spite of the use of gunpowder and vinegar the stench was so great that many of the workmen were seized with fever, and others had to continue the gruesome work. By a strange chance, on the very morning that Marie

Antoinette's sufferings came to an end on the Place tie la Revolution, the body of another unfortunate queen again saw the light of day-it was on the 16th of October that the body of our Queen Henrietta Maria, who had died in 1669, was taken from its coffin and added to the ghastly heap in the ' ditch of the Valois,' as the pit into which these royal remains were hurled was called; that of her daughter, the once ' Belle Henriette,' came next ; and then in quick succession the bodies of Philippe d'Orleans; that of his son, the notorious Regent ; of his daughter, the no less notorious Duchesse de Berri; of her husband, and half-a-dozen infants of the same family. On the same day a coffin was cautiously opened. This was found at the entrance of the royal vault (the customary position for that containing the latest deceased king), and contained the remains of Louis *le bien aimé.* No wonder that the body-snatchers hesitated before withdrawing the corpse from its enclosure, for it was remembered that Louis had perished of a most terrible illness, and that an undertaker had died in consequence of placing the already pestilent corpse in its coffin. Consequently, it was only on the brink of the ditch that the body was removed and hastily rolled over the edge; but not without the precaution of discharging guns and burning much powder, and even then the air was terribly tainted far and near.

"I turn the page, and find that we are only in the thick of all these dead men's bones and uncleanness, for the Republican Resurrectionists began by the Bourbons and had still to disentomb all the Valois, and further back, up to the Capetian line, and are not content until the almost legendary remains of Dagobert and Madame Dagobert reappear. Suffice it to add, that after Louis the Well-Beloved had been disposed of, came in succession, like the line of royal ghosts seen by Macbeth, Charles V., who died in 1380, whose body was one of the few well preserved, and was arrayed in royal robes, with a gilt crown and sceptre, still bright; that of his wife, Jeanne do Bourbon, who still held in her bony hand a decayed distaff of wood; Charles VI. with his queen, Isabeau de Bavière; Charles VII. and his wife, Marie d'Anjou; and then Blanche de Navarre, who died in 1391. Charles VIII., of whom nothing but dust remained; Henri II., Catherine de Medicis, Charles IX., and Henri III. were disinterred on the morning of the 18th ; ' after the workmen's dinner,' Louis XII. and his queen; and among other less interesting royal remains, the bones of Hugues, Comte de Paris, father of Hugues Capet. And so on the work went, till one tires even of the details of the preservation of this or that king and queen. Can anything be more shocking than to know that all the horrors of decay and decomposition will remain even after two or three centuries have passed over the lifeless form, and that, supposing one has the ill-luck to be thus coffined and one's body removed, ' a black fluid, emitting a noxious smell,' will run from out our last home, as was the case with those royal remains during that hot summer month at St. Denis in 1793 ? " - LORD RONALD GOWER in *Vanity Fair.*

Who, after reading such instances, can doubt that it is infinitely better that the dead should be quickly resolved into white and odourless ashes than subjected to insult and degradation even much less shocking than the cases mentioned in the foregoing pages? Some pretend that they do not care what becomes of their bodies after death, but a healthier feeling would make us determine that all such horrors, as disgraceful to the living as disrespectful to the dead, should be impossible now and for ever.

A CONTRAST: BURIALS IN CHINA AND JAPAN.

The following note has been sent me by Mr. Manes, who has recently spent several years in China and Japan. It throws some light on the question treated of in the previous pages, in the I comparison between two populous countries, one practising burial and the other cremation:

"In the country, near Shanghai, the land is a continuous graveyard. Everywhere, almost in every field, are graves in mounds of earth, or coffins standing exposed on four legs. I believe these remain for some time exposed, and are afterwards buried or set on the ground, and a large mound piled over them, two feet to five feet high and seven feet through. All round the walls of Ichang is this graveyard, notwithstanding that the land for agricultural purposes is valuable, and there is a dense population. There are always dozens of dogs in these cemeteries. I saw once, at Ichang, these brutes devouring the body of a boy, who had been buried a day or two before in a coffin not sufficiently strong, and with only a few stones put on the top of the lid. Many such horrible sights are seen by travellers in various parts of China.

"I saw, just outside the town of Chinkiang, on the river Yangtse, about twenty coffins stacked on the top of each other, the coffins being only a few rough boards nailed together. The place was too horrible for anyone to go near. There also are low hills of considerable extent, covered with graves of men who fell in the Taiping rebellion, each marked by a little mound of earth, which is covered with rough grass; no cultivation is attempted in the place. There are also old mandarins' or high officials' graves in this neighbourhood, which take up more space. The Ming tombs at Nangkin, where monster stone figures are set up on each side the road leading to the tombs, may be mentioned. There are smaller ones at old warriors' graves, with men, horses, elephants, lions, &c., in stone, guarding the path to the graves of the old rulers or warriors, and often taking up an enormous space of valuable land that is uncultivated now, and the home of pheasants and hog-deer. At

Cremation and Urn-Burial; or, The Cemeteries of the Future

Ichang I noticed a graveyard of several miles extent, and of the most valuable land for agriculture. Not a tree or bush was to be seen, of any size, except at a temple.

"My impressions of China are the reverse of the pleasant ones I have of Japan. It is, in fact, so far as I saw it, a sad and unpleasant country, and is to a great extent made so by the very inefficient and disgusting modes of burial one is there compelled to witness in travelling by the roadsides or in the fields. It is also a most costly plan to the country, as it prevents much of the choicest land in it from producing food, or beautifying the land near the cities with trees or parks.

"The Japanese, on the contrary, burn their dead in all cases, and while they thus save their land for the use or pleasure of the living, their cemeteries are really beautiful places. Sometimes they are placed in a lovely valley, shaded by enormous pines, and sometimes on little lawns or ledges on hillsides. Usually each family using the cemetery has a small square of ground allotted to it in which the ashes are buried.

"There is, of course, a great saving of land as compared with the Chinese, or even with our own method. Over the buried ashes a stone, often beautifully cut, containing the name of the family or individual, while vases for flowers and lamps are frequently seen near the graves in these beautiful and in no way offensive cemeteries. The evergreen bushes used to plant in these cemeteries are Ilicium religiosum, the Tea-shrub, Camellias, and Euryia japonica. I have seen specimens of the Maiden Hair tree or Ghinko (Salisburia) in these cemeteries. In the principal ones, too, may be seen noble specimens of the Umbrella pine and other rare trees. This desirable result is attained notwithstanding the fact that the Japanese mode of cremation is a very imperfect one, much more so than it need be. I speak of what I saw in villages; but in some of the cities a better system is in use. The Japanese are firmly persuaded of the merits of their system.

We have now had some evidence of the great need for burial reform, and of the state, so often shameful, of cemeteries in many different lands. The ideas set forth in the first part of this book are printed in the hope that all who cherish the memory of their dead may be led to consider the many evils of the present system, and that they may help to save us from the danger, the horror, and the degradation of the grave. It is for the most advanced and cultivated of the great nations of the West to lead the way in this essential reform, called for in the interest of the Living; of beauty of open spaces in cities; respect for the memory of the Dead, of Art, and of natural beauty.

AN ACCOUNT OF THE FIRST CREMATIONS IN ENGLAND IN MODERN TIMES.

ONE of the few present at these, I say something of them here, as the history of a separate and initial act of this kind may serve to throw light on the present state of burial in England, and may be helpful to those who wish to escape from its sickening horrors, even before there are public or recognised aids to doing so.

On Sunday evening, the 8th October, 1882, the body of Mrs. Hanham, wife of Captain Hanham, was reduced to ashes by fire at Manston House, in the county of Dorset. The following evening, the 9th of October, the body of Lady Hanham, wife of the late Sir James Hanham, Bart., of Dean's Court, in that county, and mother of Captain Hanham, was also decomposed by fire. Mrs. Hanham died in July, 1876, of cancer; Lady Hanham in June, 1877, in her ninetieth year. Mrs. Hanham expressed to her husband and various friends her wish that her body should not be buried, but reduced to ashes in this manner, and Lady Hanham desired that hers should share the same lot as that of Mrs. Hanham. Captain Hanham, her only surviving son, respecting these wishes, determined to carry them out in the face of all difficulties. These are numerous, owing to the fact that no public body exists in this kingdom which carries out cremation, and those who desired to execute the wishes of their relations in such a case were driven to seek aid in foreign countries at an amount of trouble and expense which made it impossible for most.

The cremations were carried out in a simple and inexpensive furnace, not only without any nuisance to the neighbourhood, but without the slightest unpleasantness to those who stood within two feet of the white flame which promptly resolved the bodies to their harmless elements. Though effected under many difficulties, not one of which need occur if the practice were organised amongst us, the act was well and quickly done in each instance, nothing being left but perfectly calcined bones. The fragments of the larger ones looked like frosted silver, and they broke at a touch. I gathered the ashes of each body and placed them in a large china bowl, in which they will remain until urns of an improved form are ready; then they will be moved to the mausoleum among the trees on the lawn.

Compared with the contents of such Roman and other urns as I have seen, the ashes are greater in amount and much more perfectly preserved. This was owing to complete and quick combustion, and to the body being kept from direct contact with the fire. Every part of the bony structure is represented in the ashes, but without any definite form which would make them recognisable to any but experts. In size the remains vary from pieces 1½ inch long to ashes and fine dust.

Each body was, since decease (five and six years ago respectively), encased in a strong elm coffin, and that in a lead one. The lead was only adopted because the bodies were placed on a stand in the mausoleum, and to prevent the violation of sanitary laws. The coffins, lead and all, were placed in the furnace on firebrick and iron plates, which allowed the flames to play freely up, but prevented the ashes from falling into the furnace below. Thus the shells had to be consumed before the bodies, compelling the use of greater heat and longer time than usual, so adding another obstacle. The lead soon ran through the furnace into the ashpits, and the white flames played round the strong elm shell, until that fell at white heat over the body, of which, about one hour afterwards, only the ashes remained.

The crematorium was made in a simple and effective manner by Mr. Richards of Wincanton, in Somerset, whose hands were, however, tied by the conditions first laid down to him. The plan was to burn the bodies in the vault of the mausoleum, so as to avoid removing them, and also for the sake of avoiding idle curiosity or interference, but the lower chamber was only 12 feet in diameter, thus making a long side opening necessary instead of an end one, and weakening the contrivance in various ways. But before the time of trial approached it was feared that the heat and other difficulties would make the operation doubtful, and therefore it was determined to erect the furnace in an orchard adjoining the lawn, surrounded by a temporary building. In this success was complete.

The furnace, such as it was, however, deserves a few words as the first ever used in England, and one which, though rude, did its work thoroughly. The furnace was rectangular in shape, the body of brickwork 8 feet long, 7 feet 6 inches high, and 4 feet 6 inches in breadth. The two ends and back were carried up in solid brickwork, the other side or front being where all entries and firing were effected. On the ground was the ashpit, which is cleared by four firebrick doors in a row. Immediately above the ashpit is the grate, which is fed by five holes cast in fireclay, and supported on the brickwork on which the ashpit doors are set. These holes are fitted with stoppers, being firebricks with iron handles about 9 inches square and 2 inches thick. Along the top of these upper holes rests a vertical cast-iron frame, 7 feet long and 2 feet high, which forms the entrance to the consuming chamber. Directly above the fire are firebrick arches about 6 inches apart and a foot wide, the tops of which are level with the bottom portion of the iron frame. To fill these spaces between these arches flat iron plates are placed, resting one end on the level of the lower part of the entrance to the consuming chamber, the other in the brickwork opposite. Both arches and plates are across the grate. The flames come up between the arches and curl round the iron plates freely, while the ashes could not fall to the fire below. The consuming chamber is arched over, and three holes fitted with dampers cut in the top at equal intervals. These are the communication with the flue which runs along the whole length of the top and discharges the smoke into the chimney raised on a brick platform of its own, and joining at the back of the building. The chimney is wrought-iron, 16 feet high and 14 in diameter, the first 8 feet being lined with clay pipes. It was found that ironwork in the furnace anywhere was a mistake, the iron plates being consumed by the intense heat. It would be easy to replace such ironwork as was used with fireclay plates.

As an instance of the harmless way in which the process may be carried out, it may be stated that the women servants of the house came out in the dark on both occasions, stood around, and even looked into the furnace, without any unpleasant sensations. If in so simple a beginning, in an untried and rudely put together apparatus, such success is attained, it is needless to say that the ceremony might easily be made the most beautiful and inoffensive of all.

Among the few who witnessed the process in each case were Dr. Comyns Leach, Medical Officer of Health for the Sturminster District; Captain Hanham, husband of Mrs. Hanham, and youngest son of Lady Hanham; Mr. J. C. Swinburne-Hanham, son, by her first husband, of Mrs. Hanham; Fleet- Surgeon Edney; Messrs. Stickland, Swetman, Day, and Harris, trusted helpers, who assisted in carrying out the work; and the writer.

It is as well to tell here, in Captain Hanham's own words, the origin of the wish to avoid the common graveyard in the cases in question:

"Manston House is situated on the bank of the river Stour, and its grounds surround the church and its graveyard. The river Stour frequently overflows its banks, and on some such occasions the water is within 8 inches or a foot of the surface of the graveyard. This graveyard, having been in use some hundreds of years, is full of bones. My predecessor lowered the graveyard considerably, throwing the earth, &c., over the grounds of Manston House, and filling up a depression once a pond. When I first resided in Manston, the rector was the Rev. G. F. St. John (he was rector of the parish forty-seven years). Soon after, 1852 or 1853, the sexton having prepared an open grave for the reception of a body which was to be buried in the afternoon, I observed a dealer in rags and bones named Porter' in the graveyard, having a bag on his shoulder. Mentioning this circumstance to the rector, asking him how it was that a relative of Porter's was to be buried in the parish, as they did not belong to it, he became excited, saying, ' That rascal there again. He has been there many times before with the object of collecting the bones thrown out of the grave, which he sells!'

"I made a voyage to the Pacific in the yacht *Themis* in 1864, returning in 1866. Whilst at Monte Video, a friend residing there asked me to attend a funeral. I did so, and there saw the body of the deceased person borne to a cemetery, the procession halting opposite a kind of catacomb. Here the lid was removed, the body of deceased exposed dressed in his usual clothes. A quantity of quicklime was then thrown into the coffin, lid replaced, and the whole thing hoisted up in a kind of pigeon hole. Asking my friend what was the next move with these remains, he took me to another part of the cemetery, where he showed me a most disgusting sight, namely, thousands of bones, *debris* of coffins, &c., heaped up inside a boarding or species of barn, which he told. me was the resting-place when the pigeon holes were cleared out, which occurred when the supply for room in them exceeded the demand. I believe a register was kept of the dates, and the oldest inhabitants of the holes were the first made to leave.

"I left the island of Tahiti, having previously visited the islands of Hawaii, and on the 6th January, 1866, my wife, Josephine Ida Dodson Hanham, having been an invalid for many years, died not far from the island of Oparo, in the Pacific Ocean, about 4000 miles from Valparaiso, which was to be our next port. The crew did not like a voyage with a dead body on board, but on my informing them that they might leave the yacht then, or at any other time or place, but that certainly I and the body would return in the yacht, I heard no more on the point. The body was landed at Weymouth, in September, 1866, conveyed to Manston, and borne to the vault by the crew, my only child, and the late Mr. Mark Philips, her guardian, being present. My wife had often expressed her desire that her remains should be near Manston House and the garden she loved, but had a dislike to the graveyard on account of its saturation with water. Bearing this in mind, I purchased from the rector for £10 the right to construct a vault outside, but adjoining my private aisle in the church. This vault was so well made that, on testing it, it held water, and therefore it was assumed it would keep out water. But when my only child, Maud Phelips Agatha, died, in 1869, the vault was reopened, when there was found 19 in. of water which had percolated through the arch of the vault. The water was bailed out, and my little girl placed by her mother's side. I then recalled vividly a wish my late wife once expressed in Hawaii: ' When I die, I wish I could be burnt instead of buried'. It was, alas! too late, as the body was in the parish graveyard, and in the water to which she had such a repugnance.

"In January 7, 1867, my old friend, the Rev. George Frederick St. John, died in my arms in this house of typhoid fever, he having requested to be moved here that he might be close to me. Many years since a vault had been prepared for him in the graveyard at Manston by Lady Shelley, at the time of the decease of her first husband the Hon. Charles St. John, brother of my friend. Round the vault are high iron railings, and Lady Shelley has from the demise of her first husband to the present time charged my gardener to look after the flowers and creepers in his spare time. Here is always to be seen some flower every day in the year. To prevent the destruction of these, an excavation, about 9 feet square and about 2 or 4 feet deep, was made outside the vault, so that a hole might be made under the plinth (stonework) on which the iron railings rested, to allow the coffin to be slid inside the vault. The day on which he was buried the snow fell heavily, and rain the night before. The water rose rapidly in the vault, which was at a greater depth than the external hole, and as the coffin was pushed into its place it went down with a splash into the deep and foul water!

"I married my last wife, the widow of the late Major John Swinburne in 1868. What I have narrated here was on more than one occasion a subject of conversation, and she made me promise soon after we married that I would have her body cremated if I survived her, she promising to do the same for me should I die first. As she was some eight years younger than myself, and apparently enjoying the best of health, I little thought the active part would fall to me, and I gave her a list of names of those I thought would assist her at the right time. Fate decided otherwise. A fatal disease having been discovered in February, 1876, she died in July following at Brighton. I at once resolved that nothing I could do to keep my promise should be left undone. Feeling if the body were once buried I should lose my control over it, and being desirous at the same time that in all my acts I would obey the law and give no rightful cause of offence to anyone, I had the body placed in a wooden shell and that in lead. Within forty-eight hours the body was at Manston, and placed under a canopy in the conservatory. As It knew I should have to leave home before all I desired could be effected, and not thinking this plan secure, I set to work to erect a mausoleum as a temporary resting-place until cremation, and afterwards for the urns. The completion of this occupied the greater part of a twelvemonth, and within a few days of its finish my mother, who was residing with me, died. She was much attached to my late wife, and requested me to promise that her body should share the same lot as Mrs. Hanham's and my own, and she watched with great interest the erection of the mausoleum. That such was her wish was known to Dr. Comyns Leach, who witnessed the consum-mation of that wish. At her death her body was placed in an elm coffin, and again in the inevitable lead. After a deposit for a few days in the conservatory, by the side of Mrs. Hanham, both were conveyed to the mausoleum, where they rested until Sunday evening, 8th October. During those intervening six years I was much occupied in seeking means to effect our object. I sought the secretary of a society, called the Cremation Society, which I heard had erected the much to be desired crematory at Woking. It would be wearisome to recount all my interviews and disappointments in this quarter. At one time all was arranged, and then it could not be done just yet; then it would be all ready in three weeks if I would arrange for conveyance to a station; but, though strong iron-bound cases were made and I was ready, other obstacles arose. Then I applied to the secretary of the society asking the plain question, Could an apparatus be erected at my own cost in the mausoleum? To this application, up to this date, I have not received a reply.

"In the meantime I had a friend who went to Milan, who brought such a picture of the difficulties, apparently insurmountable, in the way of foreigners desiring urn-burial. Among others, a written licence from H.M. Secretary of State for this country was said to be needed to be shown to the authorities in Italy before the bodies could be landed; and the tedious formalities to be gone through after arrival and disembarkation in that country, the difficulties, delays, &c., on its passage from one stage to another previous to arrival at Milan, then the various formalities to be gone through to various persons, made me abandon this as hopeless and above my strength. An American friend, Dr. Elsberg of New York, not only kindly made these inquiries at Milan for me, but also got all the information he could from the United States of America, where I made sure at one time the object could be effected. Then he informed me that a resolution had lately been adopted at the crematory not to permit the cremation of aliens. Knowing the lives of the strongest are limited, and I being in feeble health, anticipated the inevitable hour would arrive with my promise unfulfilled, and therefore decided to take the matter into my own hands. I sought the aid of one who has always been successful in his work, and engaged him to design the apparatus, which has fulfilled my most sanguine expectations. I only hope that those I leave behind, who have promised to dispose of my body in the way I approve of, may not have a tithe of the difficulty that I had to encounter.

With the view of avoiding some of the preliminary difficulties, the bodies were not buried, but kept in a strongly-built mausoleum of good design in the grounds. It was essential to the control of the final operation that the bodies should not be buried, and this led to the erection of a mausoleum. The building, though not large, is of the most massive and enduring character, the solid walls of the vault being 3 feet and those of the superstructure 2 feet thick, composed, as are also the ceiling and floor of the vault and the principal dome, of cement concrete. The concrete is formed of Portland cement from Portsmouth, gauged with washed grit from Moreton, and mixed with flint gravel found in the neighbourhood. This gravel was washed five times, upon a platform built out into the river near at hand, until it was free from all impurity; the result being a conglomerate, hard and imperishable as granite, and perfectly impervious to wet.

Owing to the proximity of the river Stour, and the pervious nature of the gravel soil, the site of the mausoleum is liable not only to be flooded on the surface, but also to be saturated by any rising of the water; and it therefore required some ingenuity so to construct the floor of the vault as to resist the combined action of damp and hydraulic pressure. The floor is an invert, or reversed dome, the outer segment of which consists of 9 inches of brickwork in cement ; within this, hard impervious tiles are bedded in cement; then again brickwork in cement, and the hollow of the invert brought up solid and level with cement concrete, upon which is spread the smooth-trowelled cement floor. The ceiling of the vault is a segmental arch, at once light and strong, not more than 4 inches thick, but composed of plain tiles bedded solid in cement, and carefully bonded, while the haunches are filled up solid with concrete. Thus it not only forms a secure support for the tiled floor of the mausoleum above it, but is also capable of carrying a much heavier weight than will ever be placed upon it, and is at the same time both fire and water proof. Provision was made for the efficient ventilation of the lower vault by glazed stoneware pipe flues built in the solid walls, and communicating with the upper air by means of terra-cotta perforated panels, set in the frieze of the principal external cornice.

The walls and dome are finished on the outside with Portland cement stucco, and in the interior with fine London-made Parian cement, trowelled to a perfectly smooth surface. The architraves, the cornice, and the vault and eye of the dome are elegantly moulded and polished, and of exquisite whiteness. The entrance door of the mausoleum is approached by a flight of steps of solid wrought Pennant stone. The folding doors are of East Indian teak, hung upon hinges of brass. The dome is crowned by an octagon lantern, the columns of which are of polished Cornish granite, the caps and bases of white marble, the entablature of white Mansfield (Nottinghamshire) stone, and the smaller dome is cut in solid yellow Mansfield stone. The whole is finished by a ball and Latin cross, pointing to the skies, of the purest Pantelic marble, highly polished. The interior is finished in a permanent and beautiful manner, but without excess or doubtful taste in ornament or decoration. The building stands upon a level plateau of smooth shaven turf, a terrace raised at an angle of 45 degrees forming the plinth of the building; and the whole is surrounded by a "ha-ha, or sunk fence, 64 feet by 44 feet, faced with solid masonry of Henstridge stone.

From the observations made here, a few words may be written as to some points to bear in mind in the construction of future crematoria. Ease of passing in body at end of flame-chamber; simple good design of covering building-no kind of decoration or ornament, in the ordinary sense, being attempted, except what comes from good proportions, form, and material. Easy way of withdrawing ashes, a contrivance which would serve to carry in the body and out the ashes (a kind of tray, perhaps, of non-combustible metal ?). If the fire-chamber could be made in connection with some temple where rites were performed, all the better; and in this case the chimney might be embedded in a building so as not to be visible as a separate convenience. The lower the chimney the better, consistent with the absolute need for a heat that no organic matter can resist. There should be ample openings under roof, or in it, to secure free ventilation. Easy way of controller seeing progress of combustion without opening the furnace essential-iron or metal caps swung on pivot over holes at most convenient end, and also at side, would do. It is desirable to consider cost as much as possible, consistent with efficiency, for the sake of the poor-now oppressed by the undertaker, and his various charges, in their direst need. No iron should be used in the furnace; walks and approaches should be dry and convenient. These points refer to the crematorium only. It is needless to say that the ashes should be honoured with the most beautiful buildings we can devise. At Manston House the mausoleum is at once strong and beautiful, and it may contain the ashes of a family for a thousand years.

We who are advocates for cremation being generally adopted would be the last to desire arbitrarily to limit the disposal of the dead to the only method we believe to be free from danger to the living, which saves us from the pollution of earth, air, or water- the way truly respectful to the dead and most beautiful; but we claim the right to exercise our own judgment and action in this matter, provided we violate no law. The difficulty of detecting poisoning, the only objection to cremation which needs remark, is to be met by scientific and independent testimony as to the cause of death, precautions being taken by not permitting cremation or burial in cases where, in the opinion of those qualified to judge, there is any reason for doubt, until the doubt is removed. Meeting this one objection should lead us towards another end to be desired for its own sake-exact knowledge and record of the causes of all deaths throughout the land. This is a duty of the gravest importance for State, scientific, and many other reasons, but which is now performed, when performed at all, in an imperfect or perfunctory manner by persons interested in the case, or utterly ignorant of the cause of death.

A Section through portion of a London Cemetery.

If what actually takes place in our cemeteries were known to the public, there would be an outcry against the burial system which would soon put an end to it. This diagram gives some rude idea of what has taken place in our own day in a cemetery in South London. The ground around is being built over, and soon the cemetery will be as much "within the walls" as the old graveyards that were closed a generation ago. It may be that the system here shown will not be put a stop to by reasoning only, and that horrors or evils that all will hear of must come first. But it must come to an end some day, with five millions of people in one city, and the great cities of the world growing larger every day.

Whether, as shown in evidence, the coffins have been and are placed directly on each other, or whether separated by the few inches of soil the law requires, makes little difference in the defects of the system. Evils and confusions in the world one cannot often see a remedy for: here all is clear. Purity, beauty, sentiment, feeling, all give the same answer to those who know the facts and consider the matter. Words were never made strong enough to express the state of things, as regards sanitation or decency, which this cut feebly suggests.

MR. JUSTICE STEPHEN ON THE LAW OF CREMATION.

CHARGE TO THE GRAND JURY, AT THE CROWN COURT, CARDIFF, IN FEBRUARY, 1884.

GENTLEMEN OF THE GRAND JURY,-There are a considerable number of cases on the calendar, but, with one exception, they are of the most ordinary kind, and the circumstances attending them are of such a usual character that I shall not weary you with dwelling upon them at all. One of the cases to be brought before you is so singular in its character, and involves a legal question of so much novelty and of such general interest, that I propose to state at some length what I believe to be the law upon the matter. I have given this subject all the consideration I could, and I am permitted to say that, although I alone am responsible for what I am about to read to you, Lord Justice Fry takes the same view of the subject as I do, and for the same reasons. William Price is charged with a misdemeanour under the following circumstances. He had in his house a child five months old, of which he is said to be the father. The child died. Mr. Price did not register its death. The coroner accordingly gave him notice on a Saturday that unless he sent a medical certificate of the cause of death, he (the coroner) would hold an inquest on the body on the following Monday. Mr. Price on the Sunday afternoon took the body of the child to an open space, put it into a ten-gallon cask of petroleum, and set the petroleum on fire. A crowd collected; the body of the child, which was burning, was covered with earth and the flames extinguished, and Mr. Price was brought before the magistrates and committed for trial. He will be indicted before you on a charge which in different forms imputes to him as criminal two parts of what he is said to have done - first, in having prevented the holding of an inquest on the body; and secondly, in his having attempted to burn the child's body. With respect to the prevention of the inquest, the law is that it is a misdemeanour to prevent the holding of an inquest, which ought to be held, by disposing of the body. It is essential to this offence that the inquest which it is proposed to hold is one which ought to be held. The coroner has not an absolute right to hold inquests in every case in which he chooses to do so. It would be intolerable if he had power to intrude without adequate cause upon the privacy of a family in distress, and to interfere in their arrangements for a funeral. Nothing can justify such an interference, except a reasonable suspicion that there may have been something peculiar in the death, and that it may have been due to other causes than common illness. In such cases the coroner not only may, but ought, to hold an inquest, and to prevent him from doing so by disposing of the body in any way - for an inquest must be held on the view of the body - is a mis-demeanour. The depositions in the present case do not very clearly show why the coroner considered an inquest necessary. If you think that the conduct of Dr. Price was such as to give him fair grounds for holding one, you ought to find a true bill, for beyond all question he did as much as in him lay to dispose of the body in such a manner as to make an inquest impossible. The other part charged as criminal is the attempt made by Dr. Price to burn his child's body, and this raises, in a form which makes it my duty to direct you upon it, a question which has been several times discussed, and which has attracted some public attention, though, so far as I know, no legal decision upon it has ever been given-the question, namely, whether it is a misdemeanour at common law to burn a dead body instead of burying it. As there is no direct authority upon the question, I have found it necessary in order to form an opinion to examine several branches of the law which bear upon it more or less remotely, in order to ascertain the principles on which it depends. The practice of burning dead bodies prevailed to a considerable extent under the Romans, as it does to this day among the Hindoos, though it is said that the practice of burial is both older and more general. It appears to have been discontinued in this country and in other parts of Europe when Christianity was fully established, as the destruction of the body by fire was considered, for reasons to which I need not refer here, to be opposed to Christian sentiment; but this change took place so long ago, and the substitution of burial for burning was so complete, that the burning of the dead has never been formally forbidden, or even mentioned or referred to, so far as I know, in any part of our law. The subject of burial was formerly and for many centuries a branch of the ecclesiastical or canon law. Among the English writers on this subject little is to be found relating to burial.

The subject was much more elaborately and systematically studied in Roman Catholic countries than in England, because the law itself prevailed much more extensively in those countries. In the *Jus Ecclesiasticum* of Van Espen, a great authority on the subject, there is an elaborate discourse, filling twenty-two folio pages in double column, on the subject of burial, in which every branch of the subject is systematically arranged and discussed, with references to numerous authorities. The only importance of it is that it shares the view of the Canonists on the subject, which view had great influence on our own ecclesiastical lawyers, though only a small part of the canon law itself was ever introduced into this country. Without giving specific reference, I may say that the whole of the title in Van Espen regards the participation in funeral rites as a privilege to which, subject to certain conditions, all the members of the Church were entitled, and the deprivation of which was a kind of posthumous punishment analogous to the excom-munication of the living. The great question with which the writer occupies himself is - In what cases ought burial to be denied? The general principle is that those who are not worthy of Church privileges in life are also to be excluded from them in death. As to the manner in which the dead bodies of persons deprived of burial were to be disposed of, Van Espen says only that although in some instances the civil power may have entirely forbidden burial, whereby bodies may remain unburied or exposed to the sight of all, to be devoured by beasts or destroyed by the weather (he considers the dissection of criminals as a case of this kind), the Church has never made such a provision, and has never prohibited the covering of dead corpses with the earth. This way of looking at the subject seems to explain how the law came to be silent on exceptional ways of disposing of dead bodies. The question was in what cases burial must be refused. As for the way of disposing of bodies to which it was refused, the matter escaped attention, being probably regarded as a matter which affected those only who were so unfortunate as to have charge of such corpses. The famous judgment of Lord Stowell in the case of iron coffins (Gilbert *v.* Buzzard, 2 Haggard, Consistory Reports 333), which constitutes an elaborate treatise on burial, proceeds upon the same principles. The law presumes that everyone will wish that the bodies of those in whom he was interested in their lifetime should have Christian burial. The probability of a man entertaining and acting upon a different view is not considered. These considerations explain the reason why the law is silent as to the practice of burning the dead. Before I come to consider its legality directly, it will be well to examine some analogous topics which throw light upon it. There is one practice which has an analogy to funereal burning, inasmuch as it constitutes an exceptional method of dealing with dead bodies. I refer to anatomy. Anatomy was practised in England as far back as the very beginning of the seventeenth century. It continued to be practised, so far as I know, without any interference on the part of the Legislature, down to the year 1832, in which year was passed the Act for regulating the schools of Anatomy. This Act recites "the importance of anatomy, and that the legal supply of human bodies for such anatomical study is insufficient fully to provide the means of such knowledge ". It then makes provision for the supply of such bodies by enabling any executor or other party having lawful possession of the body of any deceased person to permit the body to be dissected except in certain cases. The effect of this has been that the bodies of persons dying in various public institutions, whose relatives were unknown, were so dissected. The Act establishes other requisitions not material to the present question, and enacts that after examination the bodies shall be decently interred. This Act appears to me to prove clearly that Parliament regarded anatomy as a legal practice; and, further, that it considered that there was such a thing as a "legal supply of human bodies," though that supply was insufficient for the purpose. This is inconsistent with the opinion that it is an absolute duty on the part of persons in charge of dead bodies to bury them, and this conclusion is rather strengthened than otherwise by the provision in sect. 13 of the Act, "The party removing the body shall provide for its decent burial after examination ". This seems to imply that apart from the Act the obligation to bury would not exist, and it is remarkable that the words are not, as in the earlier section, "executor or other party, which seems to point to the inference that the executor stood in a different position as to burial from the party having "lawful possession, and has a wider discretion on the matter. I come now to a series of cases more clearly connected with the present case. As is well known, the great demand for bodies for anatomical purposes not only led in some cases to murders the object of which was to sell the bodies of the murdered persons, but also to robberies of churchyards by what were commonly called "resurrection men . This practice prevailed for a considerable length of time, as appears from the case of R. *v.* Lynn (2 T. R. 738) decided in 1788, forty-four years before the Anatomy Act. In that case it was held to be a misdemeanour to disinter a body for the purpose of dissection, the court saying that common decency required that the practice should be put a stop to, that the offence was cognisable in a criminal court as being highly indecent and *contra bonos mores,* at the bare idea alone of which nature revolted. Many also said that "it had been the regular practice of the Old Bailey in modern times to try charges of this nature." It is to be observed in reference to this case that the act done would have been a peculiarly indecent theft if it had not been for the technical reason that a dead body is not the subject of property. A case, however, has been carried a step further in modern times. It was held in R. *v.* Sharp (1 Dew and Bell, 160) to be a misdemeanour to disinter a body at all without lawful authority, even when the motive of the offender was pious and laudable, the case being one in which the son disinterred his mother in order to bury her in his father's grave, but he got access to her grave and opened it by false pretence. The law to be extracted from these authorities seems to me to be this: the practice of anatomy is lawful and useful, though it may involve an unusual means of disposing of dead bodies; but to open a grave and disinter a dead body without authority is a misdemeanour even if it is done for a laudable purpose. These cases, for the reasons I have given, have some analogy to the case of burning a dead body, but they are remote from it. They certainly do not in themselves warrant the proposition that to burn a dead body is in itself a misdemeanour. There are two other cases which come rather nearer to the point. They are R. *v.* Van (2 Den. 325), and R. *v.* Stewart (12 A. and E. 773-779). Each of these cases lays down in unqualified terms that it is the duty of certain specified persons to bury in particular cases. The case of B. *v.* Stewart lays down the following principles: "Every person dying in this country, and not within certain exclusions laid down by the ecclesiastical law, has a right to Christian burial, and that implies the right to be carried from the place where his body lies to the parish cemetery ". It adds: "The individual under whose roof a poor person dies, is bound (*i.e.*, if no one else is so bound, as appears from the rest of the case) to carry the body, decently covered, to the place of burial. He cannot keep him unburied, nor do anything which prevents Christian burial. He cannot, therefore, cast him out, so as to expose the body to violation, or to offend the feelings or endanger the health of the living; for those reasons he cannot carry him uncovered to the grave." In the case of R. *v.* Van the court held "that a man is bound to give Christian burial to his deceased child if he has the means of doing so; but he is not liable to be indicted for a nuisance if he has not the means of providing burial for it ". These cases are the nearest approach which I have been able to find to an authority directly upon the present point; for if there is an absolute duty upon a man having the means to bury his child, and if it is a duty to give every corpse Christian burial, the duty must be violated by burning it. I do not think, however, that the cases really mean to lay down any such rule. The question of burning was not before the court in either case. In R. *v.* Stewart the question was whether the duty of burial lay upon the parish officers or on some other person. In R. *v.* Van the question was whether a man who has not the means to bury his child was bound to incur a debt in order to do so. In neither case can the court have intended to express themselves with complete verbal accuracy, for in the case of B. *v.* Stewart the court speaks of the "right" of a dead body, which is obviously a popular form of expression, a corpse not being capable of rights, and in both cases the expression Christian burial is used, which is obviously inapplicable to persons who are not Christians - Jews for instance, Mahommedans, or Hindoos. To this I may add that the attention of neither court was called to the subject of anatomy already referred to. Skeletons and anatomical preparations could not be innocently obtained if the language of the cases referred to was construed, as it was intended to be, severely, and literally accurate. There is only one other case to be mentioned. This is the case of Williams *v.* Williams, which was decided two years ago by Mr. Justice Kay in the Chancery Division of the High Court, and is reported in the L. B. (20 Ch. Div. 659). In this case one H. Crockenden directed his friend, Eliza Williams, to burn his body, and directed his executors to pay her expenses. The executors buried the body. Miss Williams got leave from the

Secretary of State to disinter it, in order, as she said, to be buried elsewhere. Having obtained possession of it by misrepresentation, she burnt it, and sued the executors for her expenses. I need not trace out all the points in the case, as it avowedly leaves the question now before us undecided. The purpose was, says Mr. Justice Kay, "confessedly to have the body buried, and thereupon arises a very considerable question whether that is or is not a lawful purpose according to the law of this country. That is a question which I am not going to decide." He held that in the particular case the removal of the body and its burning were both illegal, according to the decision of R. *v.* Sharp, already referred to. "Giving the lady credit," he said, "for the best of motives, there can be no kind of doubt that the act of removing the body by that licence and then burning it was as distinct a fraud on that licence as anything could possibly be." This was enough for the particular case, and the learned judge accordingly expressed no opinion on the question on which it now becomes my duty to direct you. It arises in the present case in a perfectly clear and simple form, unembarrassed by any consideration as applied to the other cases to which I have referred. There is no question here of the gross illegality which marked the conduct of those described as resurrection men, of the artifices, not indeed criminal, but certainly disingenuous, by which the possession of the body was obtained in the cases of R. v. Sharp and Williams *v.* Williams. Dr. Price had lawful possession of the child's body, and it was certainly not only his right but his duty to dispose of it by burying, or in any other manner not in itself illegal. Here I must consider the question whether to burn a dead body instead of burying it is in itself an illegal act. After full consideration, I am of opinion that a person who burns instead of burying a dead body does not commit a criminal act unless he does it in such a manner as to amount to a public nuisance at common law. The reason for this opinion is, that upon the fullest examination of the authorities, I have, as the present review of them shows, been unable to discover any authority for the proposition that it is a misdemeanour to burn a dead body, and in the absence of such authority I feel that I have no right to declare it to be one. There are some instances, no doubt, in which courts of justice have declared acts to be misdemeanours which had never previously been decided to be so; but I think it would be found that in every such case the act involved great public mischief or moral scandal. It is not my place to offer any opinion of the comparative methods of burning and burying corpses; but before I could hold that it must be a misdemeanour to burn a dead body I must be satisfied not only that some people, or even many people, object to the practice, but that it is on plain, undeniable grounds highly mischievous or grossly scandalous; even then I should, pause long before I held it to be a misdemeanour, but I cannot even take the first step. Sir Thomas Browne finishes his famous essay on Urn-Burial with a quotation from Lucan, which, in eight Latin words translated by eight English words, seems to sum up the matter: "Tabesne cadavera solvat an rogus hand refert ". "Whether decay or fire destroys corpses matters not." The difference between the two processes is, the one is quick, the other slow. Each is so horrible that every earthly imagination would turn away from its details, but one or the other is inevitable, and each may be concealed from observation by proper precautions. There are, no doubt, religious considerations and feelings connected with the subject which everyone would wish to treat with respect and tenderness, and I suppose there is no doubt that, as a matter of historical fact, the disuse of burning bodies was due to the force of religious sentiments. I do not think, however, that it can be said that every practice which startles and jars upon the religious sentiments of the majority of the population is for that reason a misdemeanour at common law. The statement of such a proposition is a sufficient refutation of it, but nothing short of this will support the conclusion that to burn a dead body must be a misdemeanour. As for the public interest in the matter, burning, on the one hand, effectively prevents the bodies of the dead from poisoning the living; on the other hand it might, no doubt, destroy the evidences of crime. These however, are matters for the Legislature and not for me. The great leading rule of criminal law is that nothing is a crime unless it is plainly forbidden by law. This rule is, no doubt, subject to exceptions, but they are, rare, narrow, and to be administered with the greatest reluctance, and only upon the strongest reasons. This brings me to the last observation I have to make. Though I think that to burn a body decently and inoffensively is lawful, or at the very least not criminal, it is obvious that if it is done in such a manner as to be offensive to others, it is a nuisance, and one of an aggravated kind. A common nuisance is an act which obstructs or causes inconvenience or damage to the public in the exercise of right common to all her Majesty's subjects. To burn a dead body in such a place or in such a manner as to annoy persons passing along public roads, or other places where they have a right to go, is beyond all doubt a nuisance, as nothing more offensive, both to sight and smell, can be imagined. The depositions in this case do not state very distinctly the nature of the place where the act was done; but if you think, upon inquiry, that there is evidence of its having been done in such a situation and manner as to be offensive to any considerable number of persons, you should find a true bill. This must depend upon details on which it would be improper, and, indeed, impossible, to address you. I must conclude with a few words explanatory of the reasons which have led me to address you at so much length. The novelty of the matter, and the interest which many persons take in it, are a reason for going into it fully. The difficulty which a petty jury would find is avoided by my addressing myself to you rather than to them. The fact also that if I am wrong my error is in favour of the defendant is another reason for stating my views fully to you, for if he should be accquitted upon my direction there would be no means of carrying the case to the Court for Crown Cases Reserved.

CREMATION AND TUE CLERGY.

The following is an abridged report of an address to the clergy of London, delivered at Sion College, London, by Sir Spencer Wells, Bart., F.R.C.S., in November, 1888. It was followed by a very interesting discussion, which showed that a large majority of the clergy present were not opposed to cremation.

The question of the disposal of the dead is one which is of almost equal interest to clergy and laity; perhaps I may say of especial interest to the clergy of all denominations, because they have so wide a control over burial places both in town and country, and they are so likely to be asked to solve the doubts of some of their parishioners or hearers as to the choice between burial in the earth and cremation. There are some who doubt whether a return to a so-called "heathenish" custom may not be irreligious or unchristian. It would be impertinent for me to say much as to the possible danger foreshadowed by a former Bishop of Lincoln (Wordsworth), who said that "some weak-minded brethren" might have their belief shaken in the doctrine of the resurrection. But I may remind you of the reply of the best of the Shaftesburys. The late Lord said to me: "What an audacious limitation of the power of the Almighty! What has become of the blessed martyrs who were burned at the stake?" And I cannot help repeating what another bishop - Fraser of Manchester - said: "No intelligent faith can suppose that any Christian doctrine is affected by the manner in which, or the time in which, this mortal body of ours crumbles into dust and sees corruption ". And as Canon Liddon said in the pulpit of St. Paul's, "The resurrection of a body from its ashes is not a greater miracle than the resurrection of an unburnt body; each must be purely miraculous ". I will say no more on this part of the subject than to express my own conviction that the belief repeated week after week in all the churches of our country in the "resurrection of the body and the life everlasting, or the resurrection of the dead and the life of the world to come," - however this may be understood, and whatever may be the idea of the "spiritual body" which is raised in incorruption, but is sown a "natural body," - I say this belief cannot be influenced in any conceivable manner or degree by the question whether the "natural body" is burnt, or buried in the earth or in the sea, or is carried off by vultures from a tower of silence, or eaten by wild beasts. The question is really not one of religious belief or of faith, it is purely a sanitary question. And here let me quote Bishop Fraser again, he said: "This is a subject which will have to be seriously considered before long. Cemeteries are becoming not only a difficulty, an expense, and an inconvenience, but an actual danger." And the "Church of England Burial, Funeral, and Mourning Reform Association" early this year, at a meeting held in the Charter House, the master in the chair, passed the following resolution unanimously:

"The time has arrived when a determined and united effort should be made on the part of ministers of religion, members of the medical profession, sanitarians, and persons of influence generally, to put a stop, as far as is possible, to the prevalent, repulsive, and utterly indefensible practice of storing up, in the neighbourhood of great populations, vast accumulations of human remains in every stage of arrested and prolonged decay ".

And at a number of ruri-decanal meetings and conferences in various parts of the country, the following was passed as an addition to the foregoing resolution:

"That the present mode of burial in solid coffins in vaults, or in already crowded graves, is seriously and increasingly dangerous to the public health; and that the Home Secretary be memorialised to inquire into the condition of cemeteries, and the mode of burial adopted, with a view to legislation ".

This led to a memorial which was presented to the Home Secretary by a deputation introduced by the Duke of Westminster, showing cause why a Government inquiry should be instituted into the condition of cemeteries and other burial-places with a view to further legislation. The advocates of cremation support the Association in nearly all their suggestions for proposed reforms, but they do not believe that any form of burial in the earth can be free from danger to the living; and, therefore, do not stop at burial reform, but go further and advise a return to the ancient custom of cremation and urn-burial. They do not propose any compulsory system, even when death has been caused by infectious diseases; but they hope to see a voluntary preference for cremation generally arising in public opinion, and they submit that if cremation is practised under proper regulations, any objections to the custom may be answered.

I need say no more as to the religious objection. The only real objection is the medico-legal-namely, that if a poisoned or murdered body is burnt, all traces of the crime are destroyed, as no examination of the body is possible when suspicion is not aroused until some time after death. The answer to this is that much more exact certificates as to death having been due to well-known causes must be produced than are required at present before burial. Two medical men, instead of only one, must sign the certificates; and in case of the slightest doubt a *postmortem* examination must be made. One case of accidental poisoning has been already discovered by the officials at the Milan Crematorium, which would have escaped notice had the child been buried. At present a considerable percentage of the dead are buried without any medical certificate, and a still larger proportion with very inaccurate or insufficient certificates. Under proper. regulations it is almost impossible that murder or suicide can be concealed by cremation.

Before replying to the sentimental objections let me say a few words as to the sanitary advantages of cremation over burial. In addition to checking all the evils of crowded cemeteries and burial places, stopping the pollution of air and water, an immense gain may be hoped for by the destruction of the germs of contagious and infectious diseases. We never can stamp out these diseases if their germs are stored up in the earth. I have published a case where an epidemic of scarlet fever was distinctly traced to opening some graves where scarlet fever patients had been buried thirty years before.

Cremation and Urn-Burial; or, The Cemeteries of the Future

Eight years ago I read a paper at Cambridge to the British Medical Association, and I invite your attention to the following remarks which I then made:

"I must allude to one most remarkable argument in favour of cremation, which has just been advanced by Pasteur, after his examination of the soil of fields where cattle had been buried, whose death had been caused by that fatal disease known as 'charbon' or splenic fever. The observations of our own Darwin 'on the formation of mould,' made more than forty years ago, when he was a young man, are curiously confirmatory of the recent conclusions of Pasteur. In Darwin's paper, read at the Geological Society of London, in 1837, he proved that, in old pasture-land, every particle of the superficial layer of earth, overlying different kinds of subsoil, has passed through the intestines of earth-worms. The worms swallow earthy matter, and, after separating the digestible or serviceable portion, they eject the remainder in little coils or heaps at the mouth of their burrows. In dry weather the worm descends to a considerable depth, and brings up to the surface the particles which it ejects. This agency of earthworms is not so trivial as it might appear. By observation in different fields, Mr. Darwin proved, in one case, that a depth of more than three inches of this worm-mould had been accumulated in fifteen years; and, in another, that the earth-worms had covered a bed of marl with their mould in eighty years to an average depth of thirteen inches.

"Pasteur's recent researches on the etiology of 'charbon' show that this earth-mould positively contains the specific germs which propagate the disease, and that the same specific germs are found within the intestines of the worms. The parasitic organism, or *bacteridium,* which, inoculated from a diseased to a healthy animal, propagates the specific disease, may be destroyed by putrefaction after burial. But, before this process has been completed, germs or spores may have been formed which will resist the putrefactive process for many years, and lie in a condition of latent life, like a grain of corn, or any flower-seed, ready to germinate and communicate the specific disease. In a field in the Jura, where a diseased cow had been buried two years before, at a depth of nearly seven feet, the surface-earth not having been disturbed in the interval, Pasteur found that the mould contained germs which, introduced by inoculation into a guinea-pig, produced charbon and death. And, further, if a worm be taken from an infected spot, the earth in the alimentary canal of the worm contains these spores or germs of charbon which, inoculated, propagate the disease. And the mould deposited on the surface by the worms, when dried into dust, is blown over the grass and plants on which the cattle feed, and may thus spread the disease. After various farming operations of tilling and harvest, Pasteur has found the germs just over the graves of the diseased cattle, but not to any great distance. After rains or morning dews, the germs of charbon,. with a quantity of other germs, were found about the neighbouring plants; and Pasteur suggests that, in cemeteries, it is very pos-sible that germs capable of propagating specific diseases of different kinds, quite harmless to the earth-worm, may be carried to the surface of the soil ready to cause disease in the proper animals. The practical inferences in favour of cremation are so strong that, in Pasteur's words, they 'need not be enforced'."

And now with regard to public sentiment as preventing the progress of cremation, let me say that it is changing very rapidly from opposition to support. Ten years ago everyone was shocked at the proposed innovation. It was opposed by two home secretaries, Sir R. Cross and Sir W. Harcourt, but Dr. Cameron carried seventy-nine members of the House of Commons with him in support of a bill in its favour. Since the practice has been judicially declared not to be illegal, the Cremation Society of England has burned fifty-three bodies at Woking. We are now erecting a beautiful chapel there. The ashes of some of the bodies have been taken to their own parish churches and buried with scarcely any alteration in the funeral service. Others have been preserved in urns by the relatives. At New York more than a hundred bodies have been burned in the crematorium there; at Buffalo between forty and fifty; and there are nine other cremation societies and buildings in the United States. In Italy and Germany, and in Sweden and Denmark, the practice is rapidly spreading, and it can scarcely be doubted that we are now entering upon a period of rapid progress here. And if you reflect not only upon the sanitary but the sentimental advantages of the ancient custom of urn-burial, I trust that the clergy will be among the leaders of the movement in its advance. Here again I will quote from my Cambridge address, because I do not wish you to think that this is any new idea taken up hastily or without full consideration:

"As to the ceremony of burial and performance of any religious service, distinguished members of the clergy of the Church of England have shown that scarcely any alteration would be called for in our burial-service; and it is felt that, as urn-burial might be practised to any extent and for any length of time in or around churches and public buildings, in towns as well as in distant cemeteries, and without the expensive transport and ugly expensive forms of our present system of burial, men might again, as of old, rest in death near the scene of their work in life, and the restoration of the family tomb to the chapel or crypt would renew and add to the tie between the family and the church. Our places of worship and the spaces which surround them, if urn-burial became general, would be amply sufficient for the preservation of the remains of our dead for generations to come, and would enable us to convert existing cemeteries, which are rapidly becoming sources of danger to the public health, into permanently beautiful gardens. Instead of filling up large spaces with decaying dead bodies, we should have natural gardens, open lawns, pure air, fine trees, lovely flowers, and receptacles for vases, which, as well as the cinerary urns and chests themselves, might be made important helps in the culture of art. In country houses, urn-burial would lead to family burial-places within the grounds, and encourage monumental work of high artistic merit; and, in the country church, the ashes of the people might repose in the place where they worshipped, instead of polluting the earth of the surrounding churchyard and the water drunk by the surviving population, or being carried to a distant cemetery, which overcrowding must in time make only a very temporary resting-place."

A word as to the economy of cremation as compared with burial. The mere furnace with chimney need not cost £100. A pretty chapel and waiting- rooms may be erected for two or three hundred more. Half an acre or an acre of land would suffice for the safe disposal of the ashes of the dead of a large population for a century to come. The mere cost of the fuel, whether wood, or coal and coke, does not exceed seven shillings. Just compare this with the thousands of acres of valuable land now occupied by the dead instead of being used to produce food for the living. And think of the cost of each grave in any cemetery, and the charge for digging it, as compared with the cost of fuel. Then all expensive coffins become unnecessary, and the cost of an urn, or monument of any kind, depends entirely upon the wishes of the family or friends.

The advocates of cremation go quite as far as the Church of England Burial Reform Association in advocating simplicity in funerals, and in reforming the practices in cemeteries which endanger the public health. But they go further, and urge upon the clergy the advantages of a return to the ancient custom of burial of the ashes of the dead either in, or beneath, or immediately around places of worship. This may be done with absolute safety to the living, beautifying by surrounding cloisters or columbaria many a plain church, and making our cathedrals and abbeys safe and unlimited receptacles for the dead of generations to come - each one a national mausoleum. If all this is well thought over, I can scarcely doubt that both clergy and laity will before very long be of one mind in the conviction that a purer public sentiment will spread against a mode of disposal of the dead which is necessarily followed by putrefactive corruption, and in favour of the purifying fire.

CREMATION.

BY SIR SPENCER WELLS, BART.,

FELLOW AND EX-PRESIDENT OF THE ROYAL COLLEGE OF
SURGEONS OF ENGLAND.

The following address was delivered at the Parkes Museum of
Hygiene on April 25, 1885. In the absence, from illness, of the Earl of
Shaftesbury, the chair was taken by Sir Lyon Playfair, M.P.

The CHAIRMAN: You will all regret that Lord Shaftesbury is, from
the state of his health, unable to preside this evening. He has written
two letters, which I will read to the meeting:

"24 Grosvenor Square, W.,

"April 22nd, 1885.

"My DEAR SIR SPENCER,-It will not, I fear, be possible for me to
take the chair for your lecture to-morrow. I much regret it; but I feel
that I should not have strength for the duty.

"I hoped when, at your request, I accepted the honourable task, that I
should, by this day, have acquired sufficient vigour for the evening,
but it is not so.

"Would you oblige me by reading these few words to the meeting?

"I desired to take the chair, that a professional gentleman, so learned
and experienced as yourself, might have an opportunity of stating to
the country what he believed to be the sanitary benefits of cremation,
and especially to urge on the Government that, as the practice is
becoming very general, and has been, moreover, by judicial
authority, pronounced not to be illegal, the whole system must be
altogether prohibited, or placed under proper regulation.

"Unless one or the other be done, we shall live in daily peril of the perpetration of the most frightful crimes.

"I am, truly yours,

"SHAFTESBURY.

"SIR T. SPENCER WELLS, BART.

Since then he has written another letter to Sir Spencer Wells, to express his own opinion on the subject. He writes this morning:

"There can be no doubt, if we are to believe the opinions of scientific men, that there must be sanitary benefits of a very substantial character attendant on cremation. I cannot pretend to say that I know all the arguments that may be urged for or against it; but as I am sure that the bulk of the world shares my ignorance, I was very desirous that by a lecture, such as you are capable of giving, much light should be thrown on the subject. There is this argument urged on religious grounds, that it will annihilate all hope of a resurrection. I have never heard the question discussed theologically, but surely it may be met by an interrogation. What then will become of the blessed martyrs who have died at the stake in ancient and modern persecutions? But the pressing matter for public consideration - indeed, for immediate consideration-is the part which Government ought to take. Cremation has been declared to be legal by judicial authority. It must, therefore, be put under legal control or altogether prohibited, unless we are prepared to encounter a constant perpetration of frightful crimes."

I am sure that you all regret that a man so eminent as Lord Shaftesbury, both as a veteran sanitarian who has devoted a whole life to the health and welfare of the people, and who is known so widely through the length and breadth of the country for his Christian virtues and great abilities, should have been prevented taking the chair on this occasion. It is, therefore, personally to me a great disappointment that I have not found him here to-night, and in taking the chair I hope you will bear with me in the few remarks I may have to make after Sir Spencer Wells has given us his lecture. I hope we may have a full discussion, because I am glad to see present those persons who are opposed to cremation as well as those who are in favour of it; and I trust we may have the most ample discussion on the subject after the lecture is concluded. I now introduce to you Sir Spencer Wells, whose scientific eminence is so well known that it is only necessary to mention his name to ensure attention to any lecture he may give.

SIR SPENCER WELLS: Sir Lyon Playfair, Ladies and Gentlemen,- Rather less than two years ago- in May, 1883 - I stood in this place and moved a vote of thanks to a royal prince - the Duke of Albany, then President of this Museum - on the day of the reopening of this building. In the report of the council to his Royal Highness it was stated that the object of the Museum is to encourage "the practical study of all matters relating to health and the diffusion of this knowledge among the public ". And the Duke, in his address, said that most of the conditions which are necessary to health "have long been familiar to the few: one object of the Parkes Museum will be to make them familiar to the many;" and he concluded by expressing the hope "that the Museum will help materially in the dissemination of that branch of knowledge which, in the words of Dr. Parkes, aims at rendering 'growth more perfect, decay less rapid, life more vigorous, and death more remote' ". Parkes was one of my oldest medical friends. He was medical superintendent to a large hospital in the Dardanelles of which I was chief surgeon during the war in the Crimea, and both before and since that struggle I was very happily associated with him in his sanitary work; and I know I am carrying out his wishes in making known to the many what is now known only to the few-how the public health is affected by the present mode of burial, and what progress has been made since his death towards the adoption of a better mode of disposal of the dead of this and other European countries. Now Parkes, though dead, still speaks by his book, and he says:

"In densely-populated countries the disposal of the dead is always a question of difficulty. If the dead are buried, so great at last is the accumulation of bodies that the whole country round a great city becomes gradually a vast cemetery. . . . After death the buried body returns to its elements. . . . If, instead of being buried, the body is burned, the same process occurs more rapidly. . . . A community must either dispose of its dead by burial in land or water, or by burning or chemical destruction equivalent to burning, or by embalming and preserving. . . . The eventual dispersion of our frame is the same in all cases. . . Neither affection nor religion can be outraged by any manner of disposal of the dead which is done with proper solemnity and respect to the earthly dwelling- place of our friends. . . . The question should be placed entirely on sanitary grounds. Burying in the ground appears certainly to be the most insanitary plan."

These are some of the aphorisms of Parkes. He did not know, as we now do, how perfectly and cheaply cremation may be effected, and so he favoured burial in the sea rather than in land; but he said if in earth, then at as great a distance as possible, and as deep as can be. In the year 1843 Mr. Edwin Chadwick drew up a report, which was presented to both Houses of Parliament, on the practice of interment in towns; and in that report, which is still to be had at most of the public libraries, there is an enormous amount of evidence sufficient for several lectures, which has been collected together, giving the evidence as to the propagation of acute disease and certain specific diseases from putrid emanations, and distinctive instances are given of fevers of various kinds which are communicated from human remains. Then there is a chapter upon the distinctive effects which are produced by emanations from bodies in a state of decay and in a state of putrefaction; and there is a summary showing that these emanations must be and are essentially injurious to the living. There is a long series of facts showing that interments in churches or towns are essentially Injurious to the population. He shows that their removal to the suburbs is only a temporary outlet and that the suburbs have certain claims for protection from the undue multiplication of burial-places. He gives a quantity of information with regard to burial-places and the different sanitary precautions which are quite essential, so that the danger of those places should be reduced to the least possible amount. Things have been very much remedied since Mr. Chadwick's time; still, I can say that, although the evil may be diminished to some extent, it is kept up in a great many parts of the country, and the evil has been simply removed from the towns into the suburbs, where the cemeteries are being now gradually surrounded by houses and a dense population. Only a month ago, in the *Irish Times* of the 23rd March, I find an account of a meeting of guardians held at Carrick-on-Suir. Dr. Quirke, the Dispensary Medical Officer for Piltown, reported as follows: "As Medical Officer of Health of the Piltown Dispensary District, I hereby report to you that my attention has been lately drawn to the present most unsatisfactory condition of the graveyard situate in the village of Ooning. I visited this place on the 28th February, and to my horror found grave-diggers actually digging through the coffins and putrid remains of deceased individuals formerly interred therein. As they dug the grave, water rushed in from its sides, and poured with such pressure that before it was 2 ft. deep it had become inundated with water to within a few inches of the surface. The diggers were obliged to desist, and in order to complete the work it was necessary to bale out the water and dash it about the neighbouring graves. During the progress of this most disgusting business, a pestilentious stench was wafted to and fro across the graveyard, infecting the atmosphere and poisoning the air which at least over 100 individuals were compelled to breathe. In an adjoining graveyard in the same parish, I noticed that many interments had taken place where there was not 10 inches of clay on the surface, and in many instances it could be seen that the coffins had collapsed and that a poisonous and offensive effiuvium was emitted from them." The chairman of the Board to which this report was presented (Lord Bessborough) said : "This is a horrible state of things;" and one of the guardians said: "I know the graveyard well, and I have not the slightest doubt on the subject. As to the graveyard being flooded with water, I remember being at a funeral there not very long since, when so full was the grave with water that a spade had to be pressed down on the coffin to keep it from floating." Another said: "If we heard of such a barbarous state of things in an uncivilised country we would be shocked." And then Lord Bessborough said, if such graveyards are "to be allowed to remain open to the public for further interments, there should be some sort of filtering tank provided for the water oozing from the graveyard before it is used by the people, if it is as Mr. Rockett says". Upon that the *Irish Times* writes: "If the polluted water is still con-sumed by the hapless people who live in the neighbourhood, filtering tanks such as were suggested would form but a sorry expedient. A thorough and complete system of drainage would be absolutely necessary as a first precaution, and afterwards such a simple arrangement for giving the poor people water as would be approved of by a scientific man acquainted with the locality. I imagined this could hardly be true, and so I wrote to Dr. Quirke, and he replied that it was strictly true. He wrote, too: "There are seven graveyards in my district, and of *all* it may be said that they are overcrowded, save, perhaps, one ". Now, I should like to turn from this revelation of what is going on in this civilised age and country to a most interesting letter from the correspondent of the *Times* in Rome, published on the 6th of this month. In this letter I find that in the 69th year of our era, the Emperor Galba and his adopted successor Piso Licinianus were murdered. Both their heads were taken to Otho: the head of Piso was sold with his body to his widow and burnt, the ashes being finally enclosed in a handsome white marble *cippus*, placed in the tomb of the Licinian family on the Via Appia. Only a month ago workmen digging the foundations for one of a new line of houses "found a family tomb with seven handsome marble *cippi* standing in their places around it - that in which the weeping Verania placed the alabaster urn containing the ashes of her husband exactly 1816 years ago, and those wherein the remains of his father, one of his brothers, and four other members of his family were deposited ". When the owner of the property, Signor Mariani, went to see it, "all the *cippi* had been opened, and the cinerary urns which were in them had all disappeared, excepting one made of rare Oriental alabaster ". It had also been opened and was empty. "Where," asked Signor Mariani, "are the ashes that were in those monuments?" "Ashes!" replied the man, as if astonished. "Yes, ashes," repeated Signor Mariani. "Well," he answered, "in truth there were ashes, and a great many of them, but I never dreamed that they were of the slightest importance, and as they were very white and clean, I gathered them together in a basket and sent them to my wife to make lye of for her washing.' And thus have the ashes of an Imperial Caesar, adopted by Galba (as Tiberius was adopted by Augustus, and accepted by the Senate), been used in this year of grace 1885, more than eighteen centuries after his death, by a Roman washerwoman, together with the ashes of other members of his family, in whose veins flowed the noble blood of the Crassi and of Pompey the Great. But the marble monument, the alabaster urn, the sacrificial vase, the marble *cippi,* and the inscriptions are in almost perfect preservation; and had it not been for the dishonesty or ignorance of the Italian workman, the very ashes themselves - as white and pure as those which are now on the table of this room, which have been burnt in our crematory at Woking - might have remained undisturbed where they were placed by the sorrowing widow.

Turning from burial in our cemeteries and churchyards, and such places as I have described to you in Ireland, to burial in churches and abbeys and cathedrals, consider for a moment what incalculable advantages cremation would give over the present system of encasing the dead body in lead and oak, and leaving it beneath the floor where priests and people daily attend public worship, exposed to more or less great danger for months and years from the poisonous emanations which must escape so long as more than the dry bones remain. Last Saturday the late Lord Mayor was left in the crypt of St. Paul's- his body to undergo slow decay - with what amount of injury to the Dean and Chapter or to the successive congregations no one can tell. It may be small, it may be great, but dangerous it must be. Supposing, instead of placing the coffin in the crypt, at the same part of the Burial Service it had been passed into such a crematory chamber as that of which you see by the model before me might easily be erected in or under any church-supposing a body had been placed in such a crematory - that the same musical service had followed-then, after a funeral oration, or one of those eloquent sermons with which Canon Liddon keeps a vast congregation spellbound for an hour, by the time the concluding hymn or anthem or dead march had been played or sung, the silvery white pure ash - which after one short hour is all that remains of a purified body, perfectly inoffensive to the living - might be left, unchanging for centuries, in any such cinerary urn as may be seen in the British Museum, beautiful in form, exquisite in workmanship, and with inscriptions which, as historical records, are incalculably more permanent than anything of modern fashion. Think what St. Paul's or Westminster Abbey, or any of our ancient minsters, or cathedrals, or churches, might be if, instead of the coffins and their corrupting contents occupying much space-sources of danger to the living-we had the ashes only of the departed arranged in vases or urns along the sides of the cloisters, or in chapels or crypts, or beneath memorial windows, slabs, or brasses. And in graveyards and cemeteries, the same change from danger and disgust to health and beauty will ensue when the overcrowded cemeteries of to-day are converted into God's acre of the future.

In regard to the question of the resurrection of the buried or burned body, after Lord Shaftesbury's letter, which Sir Lyon Playfair has read to you, and his reference to the Christian martyrs, it is not necessary to go farther. But I should like to read to you a letter from Canon Liddon, who two or three weeks ago at St. Paul's was referring to this very subject. He quoted the following sentence from Max Muller's *Biographical Essays:* "I often regret that the Jews buried, and did not burn their dead, for in that case the Christian idea of the Resurrection would have remained far more spiritual ". This sentence and what followed were not quite correctly reported in one or two of the newspapers, and I therefore asked Dr. Liddon exactly what he did say, and he sent me the following sentences, which had formed part of his sermon: "Cremation, had it taken place, could have made no difference, except in the sphere of the imagination. The resurrection of a body from its ashes is not a greater miracle than the resurrection of an unburnt body: each must be purely miraculous. Faith in the Resurrection would have been as clear and strong if the Jews had burnt their dead as it is when, as a matter of fact, they buried them."

Now, with regard to the condition of our cemeteries, comparing what we know they are with what they ought to be, I will read to you a few short extracts from the Memorandum issued by the Local Government Board on the sanitary requirements of cemeteries. In this Memorandum the Local Government Board say it is "requisite to be observed, in the establishment of a cemetery, to prevent it from becoming a source of nuisance and danger to the living," and to avoid contamination of air and of drinking-water, that a number of requirements must be observed. I will read some of them. With regard to preventing contamination of air, they say: "Nuisance and danger to health may be occasioned, not only to grave-diggers and persons attending funerals, but also to the inhabitants of houses in the neighbourhood of the burial-ground. To obviate these risks, it is necessary that the number of decomposing bodies, in a given portion of ground, should not at any time be so great that the gaseous products cannot be oxidised into harmless substances in the interstices of the soil, or taken up by vegetation." Next, "That a sufficient depth of earth intervene between corpses and the surface". Then, "That the soil be of a suitable nature, and properly drained, the drainage water being innocuously disposed of. . . . The place of burial should be in an open situation, and at a sufficient distance from dwellings, in order that any effiuvia arising from it may be diluted by diffusion, or dispersed by the winds, so as not to find their way in an injurious state of concentration to places where they will be liable to be inhaled." Then there comes a good deal about the pollution of water, and then the sanitary requirements for a cemetery are summed up under the four headings of (1) suitable soil and proper elevation of site; (2) a suitable position, especially with respect to houses and water supply; (3) sufficient space; and (4) proper regulation and management. Then they go on to say: "It is desirable that the site of the cemetery should be in a neighbourhood in which building is not likely to take place, and also that, so far as practicable, a belt of ground should be reserved between the graves and the nearest land on which a house may be built, in order to obviate, to some extent, the risk of contamination of ground air and subsoil water with decomposing matters. Each corpse also should be surrounded and covered by a mass of earth sufficient to deodorise and destroy the putrid emanations proceeding from it; and the total amount of space should be so great that it would not be necessary to reopen any grave until the body previously interred therein should be completely decomposed." I would say that if those regulations of the Local Government Board are compared with what we know is the actual state of our cemeteries, the cemeteries would fall very short indeed of what is required. I say, from what we know, that they more nearly resemble a diagram, which I will send round to you, from Mr. Robinson's book called *God's Acre Beautiful,* which represents, in a diagrammatic sort of way, not intended to be perfectly accurate, a section from a portion of a London cemetery. He says, that if what actually takes place in our cemeteries were known to the public, there would be an outcry against the burial system which would soon put an end to it. And again: "The system will not be put a stop to by reasoning only. Horrors or evils that all will hear of must come first; but it must come to an end some day, with five millions of people in one city of the great cities of the world growing larger every day."

With regard to the *legal* aspect of the question, I may say that some ten years ago, when the Cremation Society was founded, we obtained professional opinions from Mr. Meadows White, Q.C., and Dr. Tristram, a well-known ecclesiastical lawyer. In their belief, provided all nuisance was avoided, and there was no incitement to a breach of the peace, cremation was not illegal. I had also private letters from Lord Selborne, the present Lord Chancellor, and from Sir William Harcourt, now Home Secretary, saying most distinctly there was nothing in English law to make cremation illegal. Upon the strength of these opinions we purchased an acre of land at Woking, and built a crematorium. But when it was proposed to be used, some of the inhabitants objected, and sent a deputation to Sir Richard Cross, then the Home Secretary, offering considerable opposition to it. The Council of the Cremation Society saw Sir Richard Cross in response, and pointed out to him that there would be no nuisance whatever; that there was no likelihood of there being any breach of the peace; and that there could be no religious objection to it. But he said unless we promised not to burn a human body there until the subject had been thoroughly discussed in Parliament, he would bring in a prohibitive Act. Well, we did not wish this, and therefore we gave a promise that, until the matter was discussed, we would only burn animals by way of experiment. There was a change of Government: Sir William Harcourt came into office, and we applied to him to know whether he would act on the opinion of his predecessor. He determined to do so, and considered it right, until some definite Government regulations were issued, that the process should not be carried on. We promised we would abide by the same promise we had given to Sir Richard Cross, and so the matter rested for a time. Numerous applications were made to us by people desirous of being cremated. Captain Hanham, a very old friend of mine, had buried his mother and his wife temporarily in a private mausoleum, until he could obtain permission for their bodies to be cremated legally; but at last getting impatient, he built a small crematorium in his own garden in Dorsetshire, and there the bodies of his mother and wife were burned. I believe there is a gentleman here this evening who constructed that furnace, which answered its purpose most completely. Latterly Captain Hanham himself died, and by his own desire his body was burned in the same crematorium. An account of the process was given in an interesting lecture by Dr. Leitch last year at a meeting in Westminster, when Dr. Cameron was in the chair, and when a resolution in favour of cremation was carried by a large majority of those present. I may say, in passing, that some thirty public meetings have been held in different parts of the country during the last year, of which we have received reports, at which resolutions in favour of cremation, and against burial, have been carried by large majorities in every case except one. This shows how public opinion is turning in favour of the practice. Though an old custom, it may be said to be a novelty or a revival here, and to have been only for the last ten years prominently before the public. First of all, Sir Henry Thompson wrote two articles in the *Contemporary Review,* and it was brought before Parliament by Dr. Cameron in his Bill entituled "Disposal of the Dead Regulation Bill," in April, 1884. This was moved by Dr. Cameron in a very able speech, and seconded by Dr. Farquharson, and anyone who will refer to the papers of the day will see a full report of a most able speech of Sir Lyon Playfair, who went fully into the chemical part of the subject in a more complete manner than I am able to do to-night. And what was the result? Everyone must have been astounded! The Government was against the Bill; the Opposition, led by Sir Richard Cross, was against it; and yet a Bill brought in by a private member found seventy-nine members of the House of Commons to vote for its second reading. And when you look over the list of names of those members, I will venture to say that there is not a more distinguished number of men in the House than the seventy-nine who voted in favour of the Bill nominally for regulating the disposal of the dead, but really and truly to put cremation under proper regulation. As Dr. Cameron said, it was purely permissive, and those who wished to be cremated ought not to be prevented.

Still more recently the Cremation Society have given a good deal of consideration to the charge of Sir James Stephen when trying Dr. Price, the Welsh Druid, for cremating a child on a hill in Wales. After that charge the Cremation Society felt they could no longer object to make use of their crematory at Woking; but before doing so they drew up a series of very stringent rules to prevent the possibility of anybody being burnt there the cause of whose death was not absolutely certain. If there was the slightest shadow of doubt as to a death having occurred from poison or murder, the body could not be cremated there. I will read you a note from Lord Bramwell, whose authority will be received throughout the country, and who at any rate believes that the precautions we have adopted are quite sufficient for the purpose. He says: "I am very sorry that I cannot be present at your lecture on cremation; I most heartily wish you success in its promotion. I think it is right, and, what is very rare, with no drawback. It is the cheapest, the most wholesome, and, to my mind, the least repulsive way of disposing of the dead and those we have loved. That it is legal there is not a doubt. The only objection, that murders might go undetected, I believe to be more than unfounded. You have surrounded the thing with precautions. I have heard it suggested that there are many murders which escape detection for want of suspicion and consequent inquiry. How that may be I know not, but it will not be the case with those bodies cremated under the regulations of your society." Now, I think, when Lord Bramwell says that, we may say that if our society, or any branch of it, or indeed anyone, will follow the rules we have laid down, they will certainly not run the risk of concealing a murder by burning the body. I am told that at the Milan crematorium a case of accidental poisoning was discovered in this way. The parents of a child had obtained the necessary certificate for its burial in the cemetery, but they afterwards thought they would prefer cremation. The additional certificates, however, which were required by the Cremation Society there showed that the child had been accidentally poisoned by sweetmeats containing copper. It is quite certain that if any poisoner or murderer wished to be discovered he would not go to the crematorium, where the certificates of the cause of death are so very strict; but to avoid detection he would go where the present extremely lax mode of death certificates is in operation. In his speech in the House of Commons, Dr. Cameron showed that about nine per cent. of the persons who died in Glasgow were buried without any certificate of the cause of death, and there is not the least doubt that a great number of people are buried in this country under a most insufficiemit and lax system of death certificates. So that if we did nothing more than promote a system of accurate registration of the cause of death before cremation, we should be leading to improvements in the certificates necessary before burial.

I do not think I need detain you longer than to say one or two words about what I think may be perhaps the future progress of cremation here. We have an increasing number of members, who are signing the sort of pledge which we consider necessary before they join the Cremation Society-simply that they disapprove of the present mode of burial and prefer that of cremation. The proportion in 1000 persons who have signed is about 300 professional people, 50 women, 20 clergymen, 50 doctors and medical men, and 10 military men. The numbers are rapidly increasing, and throughout the world the practice is spreading. There will be found on the table a number of copies of the transactions of the Society, in which are given figures as to the progress of cremation in the different countries. Last week it was stated that the Minister - President of Brunswick had directed his body to be cremated, and quite lately, in America, Professor Cross, the most distinguished surgeon in that country, at his own desire was cremated. There are increasing numbers in Switzerland, in Austria, in Belgium, and in Holland, and a large crematorium is about to be erected at Stockholm. There is a society in Denmark with 18,000 members, and even in Spain and Portugal the movement is spreading. Sir Joseph Fayrer, who is present, will probably tell you something about its use in India, where more than 100,000,000 of people burn their dead. I would also remark that there is very great hope that the City of London will show an example to the whole country by erecting a crematorium in their cemetery at Ilford, where some 9000 bodies are buried every year. This has been seriously discussed by the Sanitary Committee of the Commissioners of Sewers, and in nearly all cases I believe there has been a considerable proportion of the very intelligent men who compose that commission in favour of the proposal to erect a crematorium. It is not yet settled, partly I believe on account of the delay in getting better plans, and their not being quite satisfied with the experiments they have seen. I went down with several gentlemen to Woking, where we burned a horse in their presence, and converted it into ashes as pure as those on the table. I believe, when they have made all the inquiries that are necessary, we shall see the City of London setting an example to the whole country in this respect, and I trust that a full discussion of this subject will lead first to a much-needed improvement in the present mode of burial in our cemeteries; and before very long, as public opinion becomes more familiar with the idea of cremation, that we shall see, in the place of the present cemeteries, beautiful public gardens, with such urns as I have shown in photographs and engravings, containing the ashes of the departed, and permanent monuments, which may exert a most beneficial influence upon the health and morals of the people.

The CHAIRMAN: Gentlemen, it is my duty as chairman to propose a vote of thanks to Sir Spencer Wells for his interesting lecture, and to invite discussion in regard to it. Perhaps, as a scientific man, as an old professor of chemistry, you may allow me to try and remove some popular objections to this method of disposing of the dead. I think, as Prof. Max Muller has pointed out, it was very unfortunate for us that the Jews followed so much the plan of burying their dead. They did so generally, but we know that Saul and his sons were burnt, and their ashes were buried under a tree. The Jews, so far as we have any evidence in the Old Testament, had very vague ideas of a future state; they buried their dead, and that practice was followed by the Christians, who had a very distinct idea of the Resurrection. Now this practice having been followed has in the popular mind given, as I believe, an unfortunate materiality to the idea of the Resurrection, and has very much diminished our spiritual views of immortality; and I think if the public were convinced that the process of burying the dead in the ordinary way and the process of burning the dead are not only analogous, but are absolutely identical; that the final result which nature demands is the same in both cases; that in the one case it may be from three to twenty years, according to the soil, when the body is resolved into ashes, and into the constituent elements of the gases which pass into the air-if this were clearly understood the prejudice in regard to this subject would be very much removed. Science has distinctly proved that death is simply one of the conditions of life; that by the death and dissolution of generations of animated beings - not of man alone, but of animated beings-plants and animals must finally be resolved into gases which enter into the air, in order that new animated beings may be formed out of them, and new generations may come into being. Now if you will allow me, even at the risk of giving you some repulsive examples, I will show you how life and death are necessarily connected together. Take the simplest view of the case, and you will see how it follows that death in all cases produces life in a new form. Take the case of a carnivorous animal. A carnivorous animal eats a herbivorous animal; the body of the carnivorous animal immediately becomes the grave of the herbivorous animal, and the dissolution of the herbivorous animal becomes the condition for the life of the carnivorous animal. I think that Victor Hugo called carnivorous animals the sextons of nature. Take the Towers of Silence in Bombay. How do the Parsees dispose of their dead? They put the bodies on a sloping shelf in the Tower of Silence; the vultures surround the top of the tower, remaining until the mourners shut the doors, and withdraw, when they swoop down, and in half-an-hour there is nothing left but the skeleton of the person who was put upon this shelf. I think you see in this case that it is the same as in the case of the carnivorous animal - death became the source of life - the dead body became to the vultures the source of their living. But in all times there has been a strong feeling against allowing the sacred body of man to be torn, or devoured by the wild beasts of the field. Tobit got into all his scrapes and difficulties by his desire to give burial to the king's enemies; and we find it in all cases. But here is the point to which I wish to lead you- whether you bury in the soil or not, your body is devoured and eaten up by very small animals or little plants, as may be-it is not decided what; but there are constantly in the air, and in the soil in all places where there is dead matter, an infinite number of little micro-organisms, which scientific men call bacilli, bacteria, or micrococci, and these little organisms devour and break up the body, and convert it into the final and gaseous constituents. So whether it be the vultures, or the wild beasts, or these little organisms, which we know are the great means by which decay is produced in the world, in the end it is the same, and the bodies are resolved into the carbonic acid, and the ammonia and water, which are the food of plants, and which the plants remodel into organic life. The question then is, Are you to do this in an hour, or are you to do it in three years under the best circumstances, or in twenty years when the soil is bad and prevents the access of those little organisms to produce this decay and transformation? The modern Macedonian Greeks have to this day a curious practice: they give temporary burial to their dead, and they go to the grave at the end of three years and examine it. If they find that practically only the dry bones are left, they give to these dry bones a respectful and permanent burial; but if there is any flesh adhering to the bones, they believe that the body of the buried person has been converted into a vampire, walking the earth and producing great evil to the whole human race. Now that is what we do. We are continually producing these vampires. We bury our dead, but decay does not take place, and the vampires spread from our burial-grounds, attacking the population and producing disease. Now which, then, is the most intelligent plan? Modern science certainly teaches that the bodies pass into the gaseous constituents whether you bury or burn them; and the Church does not think there is any difference, or what is the meaning of the alternative phrase, "Ashes to ashes and dust to dust?" It is clear that the Church does suppose that the same resurrection takes place. How could it be otherwise? As Lord Shaftesbury put it - how could it be with the blessed martyrs who had been burned at the stake or been torn to pieces by wild beasts - those sextons of nature - these men who died in the full expectation and perfect belief of immortality and resurrection? Well, then, by the scientific view of the question, both processes are identical; for, mind, I have no objection to burial or to cremation if they are done under perfect conditions of not producing the vampires which do ill to humanity. But the more a population increases, the greater the difficulty of preventing the evils to the living from the disposal of the dead. I have seen the matter treated even in the House of Commons with a levity in some of the speeches which I very much regretted. I am sure that Sir Spencer Wells and those who advocate cremation have endeavoured to find a means of not injuring the feelings of the living. The processes are identically the same. The bodies should be burned quickly, and there should be no chance of prejudice to the living; and if all that is done I see no reason why a trial should not be given to this alternative means. It was a process carried on by many nations, and in the earliest times, as an alternative process. And since the processes are chemically and scientifically identical, we could thoroughly regulate the alternative process, making it a condition that those who prefer to be buried must be buried under conditions which were absolutely safe, which will allow the resolution of the body in the shortest time into its constituent elements, and with such regulations on both sides the merits of the two processes would soon be determined.

Sir JOSEPH FAYRER: I have listened, sir, with a great deal of pleasure, very much interest, and, I hope, a considerable amount of profit, to the very learned and excellent lecture of Sir Spencer Wells, and to the very practical, scientific, and valuable remarks which have fallen from yourself. Sir Spencer Wells was good enough in his lecture to allude to something I had said to him with reference to the process of cremation as it is practised by the population of British India. I do not wish to say that I would correct what he has stated, but I would like to make a remark or two which perhaps may modify some of it, although I am quite sure when I say it it will emphasise all he has stated. You, sir, are no doubt quite as well aware as I am that the population of our great British dependency India consists by the last census of somewhere about 253 millions of people. At least 150 millions of these people are either Hindoos or are the descendants of Hindoos, I believe-at all events, you may say of Hindoo origin; and a very large proportion indeed, probably one-half, are Hindoos of the purest caste, men of the true Aryan descent, men who claim the same com-mon origin as we ourselves do. Now I believe with reference to the highest class of Hindoos that cremation is universal; with reference to a large number of those of inferior caste, and some who are perhaps outcasts, it may be that some are burnt, but the others are buried, and the bodies of others are left exposed to the wild beasts in the open air. Then, again, there are about fifty millions of Mahometans in that country, who do not burn their dead. Then there is the old and interesting race, the aborigines, the people who preceded the advent of the Aryan race, who no doubt bury their dead, as they have done in all times-the indications of which are to be found, as they are to be found in our own country, in the stone monuments we are all more or less familiar with. Then, again, there are the Parsees, who expose their dead upon the tops of those Towers of Silence that they may be purposely torn by the birds. Their supposition of the proper mode of the disintegration of the human body is, I suppose, that it should be the means of continuing life in another phase. The Aryan who preceded the Hindoo, when he burned the body, thought he gave the best effect to the mode of separating the immaterial from the material part. So he thought that cremation was the proper way of disposing of the dead, and no doubt he thought- because in many cases these peoples, without being able to give a scientific explanation why they do certain things, at the same time do that which is sanitary-he thought, no doubt, it was more conducive to the general health and welfare of the living. Therefore I think that as far as the country of this great section of the human race goes, it is entirely in support of that which is now suggested. I take it, sir, that the objection to cremation is mainly of a sentimental character. I think that the chemical science which is so familiar to you, which you have so long taught, and which you taught to me a great many years ago, for which I owe you much, teaches that the results of the dissolution of the body by the action of fire, or by the earth or air, are identically the same, although the process in the one case may be much longer than the other. But there is still the old feeling, the old habit, and it is difficult to break with this. People cling to the old idea of the slow dissolution of the body, the "earth to earth," and so I take it they shrink from the idea of the sudden destruction of the body in the flame. But if they could, in their mind's eye, only follow, as they do probably, the process which seems to them so suggestive of violence, and could equally follow the process which goes on under the earth, I am very sure they would be infinitely more disgusted than by what takes place in the pure flame. I confess myself, although I am fully imbued with the scientific advantages of cremation, still that some of the old sentiment clings to me. Although, as far I am individually concerned, it would not matter to me in the least whether my body were placed in the earth, committed to the ocean, or burned, as I know the result must be the same, I confess - and in that no doubt there is a certain amount of weakness - that I cannot quite contemplate the application of this process to those who are dear to me. But by time and education it is probable people will become accustomed to it. Whether it will become general it is difficult to say, but I think those who have initiated this movement have done well, because from the sanitary point of view it is desirable. When you think of nearly five millions of people massed in this city, and consider how close the contact must be with the numbers of the dead constantly being buried, I think, as this becomes better known and more realised, it is probable that the present practice of burying will disappear, and I quite foresee the time when, under due precautions and proper care, solemnity, and decency, that practice will be followed by the process of cremation. I am glad to have had the opportunity of saying so much, but I would not like to commit myself any further. I would not like even now, though perhaps I may do so before long, to say that I would take part in this movement. At the same time, I certainly would not oppose it, but would rather leave it to those who know more about the subject before I press it. Although I fully recognise its excellence from the sanitary point of view, yet from the sentimental point of view I do believe it would do very much violence to the feelings of many. Therefore I think it should be approached with due caution, and I cannot conceive it could be better done than by Sir Spencer Wells and yourself. I thoroughly confess that in the three-quarters of an hour in which I have listened to him my feelings have already undergone a certain amount of change, and I am very much more likely to affix my signature to such a scheme than before I came here to-night.

Dr. CHARLES CAMERON, M.P.: I have listened, sir, with great pleasure to the lecture of Sir Spencer Wells, and also to the remarks with which you supplemented what he had to say; and the only disappointment I felt in connection with them was that, in consequence no doubt of his desire to be brief, Sir Spencer Wells omitted to touch upon one of the most important arguments in favour of cremation, which no man in London could so ably have handled as himself. You, sir, have alluded to the action of the myriad organisms on the bodies of the dead, and Sir Spencer Wells might have told us of the very important part which it has been shown those morbid organisms, spreading from the bodies of the dead, play in the production of diseases. It has been shown that many of the morbid organisms are capable not merely of multiplying in the human body and giving rise to phenomena of disease, but are also capable of living and multiplying in the earth, and of being conveyed by means of water, percolating through the soil, into the bodies of human beings, in whom they innoculate the disease which has proved fatal in the former case. That has been distinctly proved in the case of yellow fever, and in various diseases affecting animals. The discoveries of Pasteur have a most important bearing upon the question of cremation, and that from the standpoint of the safety of the living; it is of the most momentous importance that we should dispose of our dead in such a manner as to destroy those micro-organisms. Now in all the three speeches we have heard reference to the sentimental point of view of the question. To my mind the sentimental objections are entirely against burial, and the only reason why people tolerate burial is because of their ignorance. All of us have occasionally to go to a churchyard. I believe it is fortunate, or unfortunate, that the customs of this country prevent the gentler part of humanity from going to burials, for I am certain that if women were to attend our funerals they would be so utterly disgusted with what they saw, from a sentimental point of view, that they would welcome any change in our present practice as an improvement. I do not profess to be particularly sentimental, or easily impressed, but I confess that what I have seen in churchyards, on the solemn occasions of interments, has thoroughly disgusted me. I remember attending the funeral of a friend in Kensal Green Cemetery. That is a clay soil; the lumps of clay lay around the grave in masses, and in summer would have been like bricks. In that portion of the Burial Service which refers to "ashes to ashes the clerk is obliged to put his hand in his pocket and take out a handful of earth, which he has brought from another place, because the clay there will not enable him to fulfil that part of the ceremony; and to save the feelings of the people, the shovelling in of the brickbats of clay is deferred until the mourners depart. As to the medical part of the question, when it comes to the burial of the poor, if any person who is prejudiced in favour of burial on sentimental grounds will take the trouble to inquire into the mode in which our poor are buried in temporary graves and yet preserve his prejudice, I can hardly understand what his sentiments are. As to the medico-legal objection to cremation, that is the only one in which there is, to my mind, anything. The medico-legal objection appears in this country to have no weight whatever, and for this reason, that persons are allowed to bury their dead without the smallest precaution. I am not going to trouble you with statistics, but, as a matter of fact, the statistics of the Registrar-General show that every year there are buried in England and Wales, without any medical certificate or evidence as to the cause of death, as many persons as are buried in the whole of the metropolitan area in the course of two months. Now, with such a laxity in our laws, to demur to cremation, properly conducted, as likely to lead to the concealment of disease, is absolutely absurd! The Society in establishing which Sir Spencer Wells has taken so leading a part adopts the most stringent rules, I think rather unnecessarily so; but everyone will agree that it is well in such a matter, at first at all events, to err on the safe side. I was glad to see the other day that the crematory at Woking had been for the first time used for its legitimate purpose. The ceremony took place with all solemnity and decorum, and the criticism which has been made upon it in all quarters has been respectful in the highest degree. I think that augurs well for the future practice of cremation, and I am certain that as the practice becomes more generally adopted in this country and elsewhere than It has been for many centuries, the better it will be for the living as well as, I was going to say, for the dead. I might have said so truly, for if one could imagine a dead man feeling, I think he would have a preference for the speedy dissolution of his poor body to its elementary elements, as against the slow process of disintegration to which it is at present exposed.

CREMATION SOCIETY OF ENGLAND.

THIS Society was formed to promote the objects set forth in the following declaration:

"We disapprove the present custom of burying the dead, and desire to substitute some mode which shall rapidly resolve the body into its component elements by a process which cannot offend the living, and shall render the remains absolutely innocuous. Until some better method is devised, we desire to adopt that usually known as cremation."

The conditions of membership are

1.-Adhesion by signature to the above declaration.

2.-The payment of an annual subscription of one guinea, or a single payment of ten guineas.

II.

The arrangements for cremating a body at the Society's crematorium, St. John's, Woking, are complete, and are available to the public on the following conditions:

(a) An application in writing must be made by the friends or executors of the deceased - unless it has been made by the deceased person himself during life - stating that it was the wish of the deceased to be cremated after death.

(b) Two certificates from duly qualified medical men are required relative to the cause of death, one at least of whom must have attended the deceased.

These must satisfy the Council of the Society or their representative, and in some rare or doubtful case an autopsy might be desirable.

III.

GENERAL INSTRUCTION5.-It cannot be too clearly understood that it is most undesirable to convey the body in a heavy or costly coffin ; a light pine shell is the best receptacle for the purpose of cremation. There is no reason why, for the funeral service, a simple shell should not suffice, but it may be covered with black cloth at very small expense, if preferred. There is a certain fixed but ample limit for the breadth and depth of this, which is not to be exceeded. When, however, it is intended to hold a funeral service in public, and with some degree of ceremony, before cremation, a more ornate coffin may be used if desired, but it should contain the shell described, which can be afterwards removed.

When a funeral service is performed over the ashes after cremation, they should be placed in a casket suitable for the purpose.

One or more friends of the deceased may be present in the building during cremation, for the purpose of holding service in the chapel, or occupying the waiting-rooms, during the process of cremation, for the purpose of receiving and removing the ashes, if it be desired to preserve them. Scrupulous care is taken to maintain them intact and pure for this purpose.

No person is permitted to enter the crematory during the process but the officers of the Society.

A day's notice being given, Messrs. Garstin & Sons, the well-known undertakers, of 5 Welbeck Street, Cavendish Square, will provide a shell and remove the body in a hearse from any house or station within the four-mile radius from Charing Cross, to the Society's crematory.

A fixed scale of moderate charges for removal of the deceased, according to the mode of transit, the number of attendants required, the cost of shell, &c., can be had on application to the office of the Society.

The charges for the use of the crematorium, for all attendance there, and all expenses connected with the ceremony, is fixed for the present at £6, and this sum is to be paid to the Cremation Society of England on the day preceding the cremation.

IV.

Attention is called to the following "Minute of Council which has been recently passed:

"In the event of any person desiring, during life, to be cremated at death, the Society is prepared to accept a donation from him or her of ten guineas, undertaking in consideration thereof to perform the cremation, provided all the conditions set forth in the forms issued by the Society are complied with."

In consideration of the above payment the Cremation Society undertakes - on the decease of a subscriber - also to send an agent when required, without further charge, to the family residence, if within 20 miles of Charing Cross, for the purpose of supplying information and making all the necessary arrangements. By this means survivors who may naturally anticipate considerable difficulty in complying with the request on the part of the deceased to be cremated may be spared all trouble and anxiety as to the manner of carrying it into execution. When the distance is more than 20 miles, information will be supplied by letter, or an agent sent for a very moderate charge.

The necessary forms, ready for filling up, can be obtained on appl/mention at the Society's Offices, No. 8 New Cavendish Street, Portland Place, W.

J. C. SWINBURNE-HANHAM, *Hon. Sec.*

JANUARY, 1889.

APPLICATION

FROM

RELATIVE, EXECUTOR, OR FRIEND OF DECEASED.

APPLICATION

FROM

RELATIVE, EXECUTOR, OR FRIEND OF DECEASED.

———

I, (Name)...
(Address)...
(Occupation)........... ....hereby request
the Cremation Society of England to undertake the cremation
of the body of...
and I certify that the deceased expressed no objection (orally
or in writing) to being cremated after death.

A medical certificate of the cause of death is enclosed.

(Signature)...

———

NOTE.—When no medical certificate is enclosed, an autopsy
must be made and certified by a medical officer appointed
by the Society, and at the expense of the applicant or of
the estate of the deceased.

MEDICAL CERTIFICATE OF THE CAUSE OF DEATH.

MEDICAL CERTIFICATE OF THE CAUSE OF DEATH.

To THE CREMATION SOCIETY OF ENGLAND.

(Address)...............................

CERTIFICATE No. I.

I hereby certify that I attended
(Name)...
(Address)..
(Profession or Occupation).......................
aged......, that I last saw h...... on......................18......
that h......died on.........................at.......................
and that the cause of death was as hereunder written.

	Cause of Death.	Time from Attack till Death.		
(a) First.		*	*Signed*........	The First General Practitioner will sign here.
		*	*Profl. Title*................	
(b) Second.		*	*Address*....................	
		*	*Date*.......................	

This certificate must be signed by a registered medical practitioner.

* The time for each form of Disease or Symptom is reckoned from its commencement.

CERTIFICATE No. II.

I certify that I have, in relation to the expressed desire that the deceased should be cremated, carefully and separately investigated the circumstances connected with the death. I declare that there are no circumstances connected with the death which could, in my opinion, make exhumation of the body hereafter necessary.

Signed ....
Profl. Title ....
Address ....
Date ....

The Second General Practitioner will sign here.

This certificate must be signed by another registered medical practitioner.

The Cremation Society reserves to itself the right of refusing to carry out cremation in any case without assigning any reason.

Lightning Source UK Ltd.
Milton Keynes UK
21 February 2011
167916UK00002BA/98/P